Teaching Psychiatry to Undergraduates

Second Edition

Teaching Psychiatry to Undergraduates

Second Edition

Edited by

Patrick Hughes
NHS Forth Valley

Julie Langan Martin
University of Glasgow

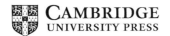

CAMBRIDGE
UNIVERSITY PRESS

University Printing House, Cambridge CB2 8BS, United Kingdom

One Liberty Plaza, 20th Floor, New York, NY 10006, USA

477 Williamstown Road, Port Melbourne, VIC 3207, Australia

314–321, 3rd Floor, Plot 3, Splendor Forum, Jasola District Centre,
New Delhi – 110025, India

103 Penang Road, #05–06/07, Visioncrest Commercial, Singapore 238467

Cambridge University Press is part of the University of Cambridge.

It furthers the University's mission by disseminating knowledge in the pursuit of
education, learning, and research at the highest international levels of excellence.

www.cambridge.org
Information on this title: www.cambridge.org/9781108925976
DOI: 10.1017/9781108921206

© The Royal College of Psychiatrists 2023

First edition published 2011
Second edition published 2023

A catalogue record for this publication is available from the British Library.

Library of Congress Cataloging-in-Publication Data
Names: Hughes, Patrick Ewan, 1985– editor. | Martin, Julie Langan, editor.
Title: Teaching psychiatry to undergraduates / edited by Patrick Hughes, Consultant Psychiatrist, NHS
Forth Valley, Julie Langan Martin, Consultant General Adult Psychiatrist; Programme Director – Masters in
Global Mental Health, University of Glasgow.
Description: Cambridge, United Kingdom ; New York, NY : Cambridge University Press, 2022. | Includes
bibliographical references and index.
Identifiers: LCCN 2022005636 (print) | LCCN 2022005637 (ebook) | ISBN 9781108925976 (paperback) |
ISBN 9781108921206 (ebook)
Subjects: LCSH: Psychiatry – Study and teaching. | BISAC: MEDICAL / Mental Health
Classification: LCC RC336 .T45 2022 (print) | LCC RC336 (ebook) | DDC 616.890076–dc23/eng/20220225
LC record available at https://lccn.loc.gov/2022005636
LC ebook record available at https://lccn.loc.gov/2022005637

ISBN 978-1-108-92597-6 Paperback

....

Contents

Contributors

Dr Seri Abraham
Consultant Liaison Psychiatrist, Pennine Care NHS Foundation Trust Visiting Senior Lecturer at Manchester Metropolitan University TPD Core training – HEENW

Dr Mike Akroyd
Consultant Psychiatrist, Clinical Director & Clinical Teaching Fellow, Derbyshire Healthcare NHS Foundation Trust

Neeraj Bhardwaj
Digital Education Manager, University of Glasgow

Dr Sophie Butler
ST6 General Adult Psychiatry, Kings College Hospital Liaison

Dr Robert Clafferty
Consultant Psychiatrist, NHS Lothian. Honorary Senior Lecturer, University of Edinburgh

Dr Angela Cogan
Consultant in Liaison Psychiatry, Queen Elizabeth University Hospital, Glasgow Head of Student Support, Sub Dean for Psychiatry, University of Glasgow Undergraduate School of Medicine

Professor Subodh Dave
Consultant Psychiatrist and Deputy Director of Undergraduate Medical Education, Derbyshire Healthcare Foundation TrustProfessor of Psychiatry, University of Bolton

Chair, Association of University Teachers of Psychiatry

Professor Nisha Dogra
Emeritus Professor, University of Leicester

Dr Neera Gajree
Consultant in General Adult and Addictions Psychiatry, NHS Lanarkshire Associate Postgraduate Dean for Psychiatry Simulation, NHS Education for Scotland

Dr Ahmed Hankir
Institute of Psychiatry, Psychology and Neuroscience, King's College London

Dr Rekha Hegde
Consultant Psychiatrist Older Adult Liaison Honorary Senior Clinical Lecturer University Glasgow Educational supervisor Core Psychiatry Lanarkshire National TPD Old Age Psychiatry Scotland

Professor Faith Hill
Emeritus Professor School of Medicine, University of Southampton

Dr Genevieve Holt
Consultant Old Age Psychiatrist, Hertfordshire Partnership NHS Foundation Trust

Katharine Huggins
University of Kent

Dr Patrick Hughes
Consultant Psychiatrist, NHS Forth Valley

Gordon Johnston
Independent Consultant (Lived Experience)

Dr Dimitar Karadzhov
Lecturer, College of Medical, Veterinary and Life Sciences, University of Glasgow

Dr Khalid Karim
Associate Professor in Medial Education, Leicester Medical School, University of Leicester, and Honorary Consultant in Child and Adolescent Psychiatry, Leicestershire Partnership Trust

Dr Miranda Kronfli
Lecturer (Teaching) in Medical Education UCL Medical School, Royal Free Hospital, London

Dr Wai Lan Imrie
Consultant Psychiatrist, General Adult Psychiatry TPD (West of Scotland); Psych Link to DME

Dr Julie Langan Martin
Senior Lecturer in Psychiatry and Honorary Consultant Psychiatrist, University of Glasgow

Professor Brian Lunn
Emeritus Professor, School of Medical Education Newcastle University, Newcastle University

Dr Amy Manley
Consultant in Liaison Psychiatry, Bristol Royal Infirmary

Dr Daniel Martin
Consultant Psychiatrist, NHS Greater Glasgow and Clyde

Laura McNaughton
Digital Learning Technologist, University of Glasgow

Zoé Mulliez
Policy and Campaigns Manager, The Royal College of Psychiatrists

Professor Jo-Anne Murray
Professor of Educational Innovation

Nikki Nabavi
Medical Student, University of Manchester, Medical Student Representative, RCPsych Committees

Dr Helena Paterson
Senior Lecturer, School of Psychology, University of Glasgow

Simon Rose
Lived Experience Educator, Derbyshire Healthcare NHS Foundation TrustHonorary Clinical Teacher, Academic Unit of Medical Education, University of SheffieldPatient Representative on Council, Royal College of Psychiatrists

Dr Kenneth Ruddock
Clinical Teaching Fellow, Department of Medical Education, NHS Lanarkshire

Dr Neelom Sharma
Consultant Psychiatrist and Honorary Clinical Senior Lecturer Programme Theme Head: Psychological Aspects of Medicine NHS Lothian & University of Edinburgh

Dr Laura Sharp
Senior Lecturer, College of Medical, Veterinary and Life Sciences, University of Glasgow

Alexa Sidwell
Senior Clinical Educator, Psychiatry Teaching Unit, Medical Annexe, Radbourne Unit, Derbyshire Healthcare NHS Foundation Trust

Dr Derek K. Tracy
Medical Director, West London NHS Trust. Senior Lecturer, King's College London and University College London

Dr Patricia Vinchenzo
Foundation Doctor, Countess of Chester Hospital NHS Foundation Trust, Chester, UK

Dr Barbara Wood
Consultant Psychiatrist in Psychotherapy, South London and Maudsley NHS Trust

Balint Society Leader and Trainer Undergraduate Lead for Reflective Practice, GKT School of Medicine

Dr Rashid Zaman
Department of Psychiatry, University of Cambridge

Dr Angeliki Zoumpouli
Consultant Psychiatrist in Psychotherapy, South London and Maudsley NHS Trust

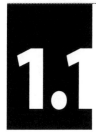

The Teacher

Dr Patrick Hughes

Introduction

We start this book with a discussion of 'The Teacher' and what that means in the context of medical education in general, and psychiatry specifically. For many, the traditional image of the teacher as an authority figure giving lectures at the front of the class persists, but in recent years there have been significant changes with regards to who delivers teaching, how this is done, and even what we are trying to achieve. Teaching is no longer delivered didactically by a handful of professors at the university, but more often by clinicians and trainees who contribute to education in addition to their clinical work. Indeed, ability to teach is a professional competency outlined in postgraduate training schemes and within *General Medical Council* (GMC) documents (Good Medical Practice, 2013). The role of 'doctor as teacher' takes many forms: formal roles at a university, informal teaching in clinics and wards, and contributions to assessment and curriculum development, to name a few (Harden and Crosby, 2000). Many medical educators don't have medical backgrounds and bring distinct points of view, diversity, and specialist expertise to the role. We believe that everyone involved in medical education should understand and employ the qualities of 'The Teacher' that are explored in this chapter.

What Does it Mean to 'Teach'?

This may seem like a simple question, but it is worth considering the following two definitions:

Teach /tiːtʃ/

Verb
1. Impart knowledge to or instruct (someone) as to how to do something.
2. Cause (someone) to learn or understand something by example or experience.

www.lexico.com/definition/teach, powered by *Oxford English UK Dictionary*

The first definition might be considered the *act* of delivering a lecture or a tutorial to students and is independent of whether any learning takes place. Within medical education it might seem reasonable to have the view that, while the audience may be diverse in terms of age and background, they are all 'adult learners', and as such the onus should be on them to pay attention and to learn from what is being offered. Even without exploring the psycho-social factors which might influence learning, we know that the brain is still developing biologically though our twenties, and this can have a significant impact on factors such as motivation. As such, although there may be a degree of truth in this idea, it is also a bit naïve to think it is as simple as that, particularly for a psychiatrist who is supposed to be an expert in such things.

The second definition may be more helpful and defines teaching as an *outcome*, with teaching only occurring if learning takes place. Adoption of this view means accepting that if the students didn't learn what you wanted them to learn, then you didn't actually teach them, regardless of how much information was in your slides. For the medical educator, adoption of this definition shifts their objective from 'I need to deliver a lecture' to 'I need to help the students understand X.' With this new objective the teacher is able to consider how best they might achieve that aim given the topic to be covered, the audience, the resources available, etc. The aim of this book is to help with that.

Shifting to this second definition opens us up to reflection on the factors that might influence a student's engagement and motivation to learn. The parallels with the doctor–patient relationship in psychiatry are worth considering. This is a partnership in which we work with the patient and provide them with the information they need to make healthy choices. When this isn't working, we may talk to the patient about taking more responsibility, but we also recognise that this may be difficult for the patient for many reasons related to their background, personality, and life experiences, and that to some extent they are acting how they have learnt to act in certain circumstances. In such cases it is necessary to then consider how the circumstances or environment might be modified to make it easier for the patient to make better choices and ultimately have better outcomes. An example might be a patient who regularly forgets to take their medication: the solution might be to arrange for someone to remind them every day; alternatively, you might provide psychoeducation about their condition and information about the medication options in order to improve the patient's understanding. Both options have their place but the point is that as doctors we do not adopt a 'take it or leave it' approach to care; we recognise that there are factors under our control which could lead to better outcomes, and the same is true of teaching. What is taught, how it is presented, context, relevance – these are all determined by the teacher and will have a big impact on whether learning takes place. There are of course other factors over which we don't have control, such as student personality, learning style, pressures from personal life, and pressures from other parts of the curriculum. Ultimately, students do need to learn to manage their own learning, but as teachers we need to consider whether the environment we are creating is making this easier for them or harder.

Lived Experience Inputs to Teaching

Gordon Johnston

Teachers do not have to teach alone or teach every element of a course themselves. Other inputs can both provide differing perspectives for students to consider and enable them to develop a wider view of psychiatry.

It can be extremely useful in the teaching process to involve people with lived experience of mental ill health at all stages as part of an extended teaching team. Their valuable input can enable greater understanding among students of the effects of living with mental illness on individual lives, thinking beyond the symptoms which can be memorised from a textbook.

Throughout this book there will be inserts like this to provide suggestions for roles that people with lived experience could play and inputs they could provide to support the teaching process.

What Else Are You Communicating?

In many ways the teaching of knowledge and skills is the easier part of being a teacher; it is certainly easier to talk about and explain. However, in recent years there has been increasing interest in what students learn from a teacher or an institution indirectly. The topics which are taught, which ones are prioritised, how ethics are discussed and considered: these all communicate something to the student about the values of the teacher and, by extension, what should be expected of a doctor and a psychiatrist. The awareness and sensitivity of the teacher to issues such as equality and diversity will also be picked up by the students and internalised. Do all your case vignettes revolve around Paul and Mary, a white, British, heterosexual couple? Are you openly critical of the curriculum, faculty, or other specialties? Mahood (2011) observes that everything we say (and don't say), every action, joke, and irritation, conveys values and attitudes to the students, whether we mean them to or not. This is often referred to as the 'hidden curriculum', and students may learn more from these modelled behaviours than from the formal teaching they receive (Mahood, 2011). Doctors may be aware of their position as role models in clinical settings, but it is just as important in the teaching role. Teachers acting as role models in the undergraduate setting can have a significant impact on reducing stigma (Martin et al., 2020) and improving recruitment to psychiatry (Appleton et al., 2017). Furthermore, how we react and respond when we make a mistake or don't know an answer can have a huge impact on the students' understanding of what it means to be a doctor and how they are supposed to act. Psychiatrists should be better than most at recognising what they might be communicating through their appearance and behaviours, in addition to what they are saying, and as such we have the power to make an important impact. Similarly, any disparity between what an institution says and does will be picked up by the students. Hafferty (1998) gives the example of a medical school with a mission statement to 'train excellent, compassionate physicians rather than the most knowledgeable physicians', but which has an awards system for the highest grades without any recognition of skills related to empathy or compassion.

'Know Thyself'

– Temple of Apollo at Delphi

Just like the students and patients described earlier, teachers and doctors are human beings with their own backgrounds, perspectives, and biases. If we are to have any control over the hidden curriculum it is essential to be aware of this as, unchecked, they can easily seep into and colour our teaching without us realising. While this is true for all teachers, it is worthy of specific mention when it comes to teaching psychiatry. Mental illness as a concept can be difficult to pin down, and we use a number of different models to conceptualise and explain symptoms. Some of these are more comfortably couched within a biomedical model, for example, Alzheimer's disease, but others are more helpfully considered in psychosocial terms – for instance, symptoms arising due to an individual's difficulties functioning in a specific social setting, as we see with the personality disorders. Going beyond this, we know that there are groups of conditions specific to certain cultures – so-called Cultural Concepts of Distress – where groups of symptoms have been observed and explained using local models for mental illness. In many cultures across the world, it is not uncommon for psychiatric symptoms to be explained as being caused by magic or possession by evil spirits, and it would be very arrogant of western psychiatrists to dismiss these models of mental illness as simply 'wrong'. The point is that it is important to recognise the perspective you are coming from and the associated biases that you might have, in order to acknowledge that students (and patients) may differ in their views and understanding. It would be arrogant to assume that 'I am right and you are wrong', as there are many ways to conceptualise mental illness – who is to say which way is the most 'correct'? Sensitivity to and respect for the different beliefs and cultures of others is another part of the hidden curriculum that should come through when you are teaching, and the topics in psychiatry are a rich vehicle with which to achieve this.

What's in it for Me?

Lastly, it is important to acknowledge the benefits that can come from choosing to develop as a teacher in medical education, including the development of transferable skills. Dayson and Hill (2011) discussed this as part of their medical teaching skills programme at the University of Southampton. They recognised that teaching forces us to examine and organise our existing knowledge, and that questions from students highlight the gaps in our own learning. Rather than worrying about this, they proposed that we should try to accept it. Instead of presenting an illusion of omniscience, we should aim to engage authentically and honestly with the students and participate in the process of learning and enquiry with them.

Communication skills are also vital, and a large part of the role of a psychiatrist is psychoeducation: explaining a diagnosis or a formulation to a patient in a way that they can understand, providing information in digestible chunks, and checking understanding. We aim to give them information to allow them to weigh up options and make informed decisions about their care. These same skills can be used and developed in your role as a teacher if done correctly, with clear benefits for both your clinical and non-clinical work. The ability to explain complex ideas in a way that people can understand and retain is a valuable skill, and choosing to develop as a teacher of psychiatry is the perfect setting in which to hone it.

The chapters in this book will give advice on how you can get more involved in medical education as you progress in your career.

References

Appleton, A., Singh, S., Eady, N., and Buszewicz, M. (2017). Why did you choose psychiatry? A qualitative study of psychiatry trainees investigating the impact of psychiatry teaching at medical school on career choice. *BMC Psychiatry*, **17** (1): 276. https://doi.org/10.1186/s12888-017-1445-5.

Dayson, D. and Hill, F. (2011). Teaching trainee psychiatrists how to teach medical students: The Southampton model. In T. Brown and J. Eagles (eds.), *Teaching Psychiatry to Undergraduates*, 1st ed. RCPsych Publications, 119–28.

GMC (2013). Good Medical Practice. www.gmc-uk.org/-/media/documents/

good-medical-practice—english-20200128_
pdf-51527435.pdf.

Hafferty, F. W. (1998). Beyond curriculum
reform: confronting medicine's
hidden curriculum. *Acad Med* **73** (4):
403–7.

Harden, R. M. and Crosby, J. (2000). AMEE
Education Guide No. 20: The good teacher
is more than a lecturer – the twelve roles
of the teacher. *Medical Teacher*, **22**,
334–47.

Mahood, S. C. (2011). Medical educations:
Beware the hidden curriculum. *Canadian
Family Physician*, **57** (9): 983–5.

Martin, A., Chilton, J., Gothelf, D., and
Amsalem, D. (2020). Physician
self-disclosure of lived experience improves
mental health attitudes among medical
students: A randomized study. *Journal of
Medical Education and Curricular
Development*, 7, 2382120519889352. https://
doi.org/10.1177/2382120519889352.

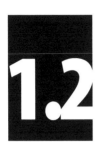

The Curriculum

Dr Julie Langan Martin

Introduction

This chapter focuses on exploring the concept of a curriculum in the context of medical education and psychiatry. We discuss the importance of the interaction between the planned, delivered, and experienced curriculum and highlight the dynamic nature of keeping curricula 'up to date'. We reflect on the importance of having a clear and transparent curriculum for both students and teachers and consider the concept of the 'hidden curriculum'. Having an awareness of the curriculum and where the teaching you deliver sits within it is important for all teachers, as this knowledge will help ensure your teaching is effective.

What is the Curriculum and Why is it Important?

In education, a curriculum can be considered as being the 'totality of the student experiences that occur in the educational setting' (Wiles, 2008, p. 2). As such, it can be considered as a wide term extending beyond the core syllabus. The word 'curriculum' has its roots in Latin, where it means 'track' or 'the course of a race'. Therefore, the curriculum can be thought of as extending throughout the undergraduate journey.

In many medical schools, psychiatry is introduced into the curriculum in the penultimate years. This presents many challenges as, by this time in training, medical students may have fixed views about which specialities are important and prestigious. This can inadvertently lead to issues with stigma and negative attitudes about psychiatry, psychiatrists, and even the patients we treat. Therefore, careful planning of the curriculum is essential to ensure that all specialities are given the recognition they require to ensure that all graduates are equipped with the knowledge, skills, and attitudes to be a good doctor.

Having an awareness of where the teaching you deliver sits within the psychiatric curriculum can be helpful for the educator. This awareness allows the teacher to design the learning experience to fit the needs of the students. For example, students who have had little prior experience of psychiatry, or who had large gaps between psychiatric teaching sessions, will benefit from focussed reminders about key skills and knowledge: mental state examination, psychiatry-specific terminology, etc. Ensuring these key concepts and skills are understood by students will make your teaching more effective.

The curriculum itself can be considered to have several parts: the explicit, the implicit (including hidden), the excluded, and the extra-curricular (Prideaux, 2003). The explicit curriculum can be considered as the planned learning that the teacher wishes to deliver. The implicit or 'hidden' curriculum (which is further detailed below) is thought to be that which is *actually* learnt in the learning environment and will be impacted by conscious and

> **Box 1.2.1 Three Levels of the Curriculum**
> 1. **The Planned Curriculum:** what is planned for the students,
> 2. **The Delivered Curriculum:** what is organised by the curriculum development team and delivered by the teachers, and
> 3. **The Experienced Curriculum:** what the students actually learn.

unconscious factors, such as teacher's attitudes and behaviours. The excluded curricula, or 'null curricula', includes that which is not taught; finally, 'extra-curricular' refers to that which is not included in the explicit core curriculum and can be taught during additional learning opportunities. Curricula can also be thought as being delivered at three levels (see Box 1.2.1).

The curriculum, therefore, is key to medical education, and some argue that success in achieving educational goals relies heavily on the quality of the curriculum (Yamani, Changiz, and Adibi, 2010). The curriculum is often underpinned by a set of values and beliefs about what the student *should* know. As such, it is reliant on those who deliver it. In some cases, teachers may support underlying values that are no longer relevant. This can lead to the so-called 'sabre-toothed tiger' curriculum, which is based on the idea of teaching out of date or extinct values and beliefs (Prideaux, 2003). A modern medical curriculum should be underpinned by values that are modern, relevant, and will enhance health-service provisions. Therefore, the curriculum should aim to be flexible, dynamic, and responsive to changing values and expectations in both education and the health service. Ensuring the curriculum is up to date and relevant can be challenging, and often a good place to start is ensuring you have a clear curriculum map and to undertake regular curriculum reviews.

High-quality psychiatric teaching within the medical curriculum is essential not only for the future of psychiatry but also for all future medical care and treatment. While there is 'no health without mental health', all medical students should be equipped with the knowledge, skills, and attitudes to recognise, assess, and diagnose mental illness, recognise psychiatric emergencies, know when to seek senior advice, and referral to specialist psychiatric services (Royal College of Psychiatrists, 2017). Having a curriculum that is relevant and up to date is a key part of this.

Curriculum Design and Delivery

In the United Kingdom, the General Medical Council (GMC) sets the standards required of medical training organisations and the outcomes that students and doctors in training should achieve. They structure the outcomes for graduates across three domains: professional values and behaviours, professional skills, and professional knowledge (Outcomes for Graduates, GMC, 2019) and highlight a number of key principles that should underpin the curricula (Excellence by design: standards for postgraduate curricula, GMC, 2017). These are detailed in Table 1.2.1.

Psychiatry and psychiatrists are well placed to allow students to meet these outcomes, especially as all these principles underpin psychiatric care and treatment. Therefore, ensuring medical students are exposed to high-quality psychiatric teaching, which is embedded, but accessible and visible within the medical curriculum is essential. While all doctors have a professional duty to contribute to the teaching and training of medical students and

Table 1.2.1 Outcomes for graduates and key principles underpinning curricula

Outcome for Graduates, GMC, 2019:	Key Principles underpinning curricula, GMC, 2017:
Professional values and behaviours	Patient safety as the first priority
	Maintaining standards across the United Kingdom
	Encouraging excellence
Professional skills	Embedding fairness
Professional knowledge	Ensuring that the current and future workforce and service needs are met

doctors in training, the curriculum upon which the teaching is based should be relevant to their work as doctors and needs careful consideration and planning (Royal College of Psychiatrists, 2017).

The Core Curriculum in Psychiatry, published by the Royal College of Psychiatrists (RCPsych), aims to ensure 'that all future doctors in every speciality respect and support the delivery of high-quality psychiatric care across the lifespan, and encourage motivated students to consider a career in psychiatry' (p. 1). It is a helpful starting point when considering what should be covered within an undergraduate medical course.

Learning from People with Lived Experience

Gordon Johnston

The doctor–patient relationship sits at the core of the psychiatric process and must therefore be a fundamental part of the curriculum. One part of the development of the knowledge, skills, and attitudes of the student could usefully include reinforcement of the notion of learning from people with lived experience.

Students should be encouraged to think not only of medical conditions and diagnoses but also of the impacts that both illness and treatment can have on the patient. The most direct, and most powerful, medium for this message is to hear it straight from those with lived experience as a core component of the curriculum. Talks, discussion sessions, and seminars can all be planned as varied methods of enabling lived experience input and promoting dialogue with students.

The Hidden Curriculum

Finally, the concept of the 'hidden curriculum' is important to consider within both the psychiatric and the wider medical curricula. While in recent years there has been much work undertaken to overview and update the undergraduate medical curriculum in terms of its explicit content, its intended learning outcomes (ILOs), its delivery, and its assessments, less attention has been paid to the 'hidden curriculum'.

The 'hidden curriculum' acknowledges that there is a difference between *what is being taught* and *what is being learnt*. Accordingly, the hidden curriculum can be considered as that which creates the difference (Rajput, Mookerjee, and Cagande, 2017). It can be further conceptualised as a set of implicit beliefs, behaviours, ideas, or values that are observed and learnt (Lempp and Seale, 2004). Learners infer these implicit messages from individual role models and group dynamics, as well as processes and structures (Mulder et al., 2018). The 'hidden curriculum' therefore cannot be standardised, written in curricula documents, or always planned for. Many argue that hidden aspects of curricula are especially important in the education of the 'professional' (Bird, Conrad, Fremont, and Hafferty, 2000) due to the time that is spent on placements and thus exposure to the predominant culture and customs. As such, the concept of a 'hidden curriculum' is not unique to medical education, and is also noted in dental (DeSchepper, 1987) and nursing curricula (Mayson and Hayward, 1997).

At times, the 'hidden curriculum' is described negatively, and some consider aspects of it to be detrimental to overall professionalism (Rajput, Mookerjee, and Cagande, 2017). Aspects such as loss of idealism (Sinclair, 1997), changes in ethical integrity (Coldicott, Pope, and Roberts, 2003), acceptance of hierarchy (Bird, Conrad, Fremont, and Hafferty, 2000), and emotional neutralisation (Helman, 1991) have been identified as negative aspects of the 'hidden curriculum'. In particular, the loss of the idealism with which so many students enter medical school has been recognised as a negative effect of the 'hidden curriculum'. This loss of idealism in students may occur in part due to increased demands on teachers' time, overload of work, and systemic difficulties in providing patient-centred care. Being aware of this and, if appropriate, challenging these cultures and customs when teaching and working is of importance to everyone.

The next chapter considers the way in which knowledge, skills, and attributes in medical education are taught.

References

Bird, F., Conrad, P., Fremont, A. M., Hafferty, F. W. (2000). Reconfiguring the sociology of medical education: emerging topics and pressing issues. In: Bird, F., Conrad, P., Fremont, A. M., eds. *Handbook of medical sociology*, 5th ed. New York: Prentice Hall: 238–56.

Coldicott, Y., Pope, C., Roberts, C. (2003). The ethics of intimate examinations-teaching tomorrow's doctors. *BMJ* 2003, **326**: 97–101.

DeSchepper, E. J. (1987). The hidden curriculum in dental education. *J Dent Educ*, **51**: 575–7.

GMC. (2017). Excellence by Design: Standards for Postgraduate Curricula. Available at: www.gmc-uk.org/-/media/documents/excellence-by-design---standards-for-postgraduate-curricula-2109_pdf-70436125.pdf.

GMC. (2019). Outcomes for Graduates: Structure and Overarching Outcome. www.gmc-uk.org/education/standards-guidance-and-curricula/standards-and-outcomes/outcomes-for-graduates/outcomes-for-graduates/structure-and-overarching-outcome#structure-of-the-outcomes.

Helman, C. (1991). The dissection room. In *Body Myths*. London: Chatto and Windus: 114–23.

Lempp, H. and Seale, C. (2004). The hidden curriculum in undergraduate medical education: qualitative study of medical students' perceptions of teaching. *BMJ (Clinical research ed.)*, **329** (7469): 770–3. https://doi.org/10.1136/bmj.329.7469.770

Mayson, J. and Hayward, W. (1997). Learning to be a nurse: the contribution of the hidden curriculum in the clinical setting. *Nurse Pract N Z* **12**: 16–22.

Mulder, H., Ter Braak, E., Chen, H. C., and Ten Cate, O. (2019). Addressing the hidden curriculum in the clinical workplace: A practical tool for trainees and faculty. *Med Teach*, **41** (1): 36–43. https://doi.org/10.1080/0142159X.2018.1436760. Epub 2018 Feb 28. PMID: 29490529.

Promoting Excellence: Standards for medical education and training. GMC Available at: www.gmc-uk.org/-/media/documents/promoting-excellence-standards-for-medical-education-and-training-2109_pdf-61939165.pdf.

Prideaux, D. (2003). ABC of learning and teaching in medicine: *Curriculum Design*. *BMJ*, **326**: 267. https://doi.org/10.1136/bmj.326.7383.268.

Rajput, V., Mookerjee, A., and Cagande, C. (2017). *The Contemporary Hidden Curriculum in Medical Education*. *MedEdPublish*, **6** (3): 41.

Royal College of Psychiatrists. (2017). Core Curriculum in Psychiatry, October 2017, Royal College of Psychiatrists Undergraduate Curriculum. Available at: www.rcpsych.ac.uk/docs/default-source/training/training/undergraduate-curriculum-2017---2021-revision---academic-faculty.pdf?sfvrsn=bc103cb6_2.

Sinclair, S. (1997). *Making doctors. An institutional apprenticeship*. Oxford: Berg.

Wiles, J. (2008). *Leading Curriculum Development*. Thousand Oaks, CA: Corwin.

Yamani, N., Changiz, T., and Adibi, P. (2010). Professionalism and hidden curriculum in medical education Isfahan: Isfahan University of Medical Sciences. Cited in Sarikhani, Y., Shojaei, P., Rafiee, M. et al. (2020). Analyzing the interaction of main components of hidden curriculum in medical education using interpretive structural modeling method. *BMC Med Educ*, **20**, 176. https://doi.org/10.1186/s12909-020-02094-5.

1.3

Knowledge, Skills and Attitudes

Professor Faith Hill

The different domains of knowledge, skills and attitudes are like the learner driving mantra 'mirror, signal and manoeuvre'. Experienced practitioners move seamlessly through the three without distinguishing one from the other. However, medical schools list student-learning outcomes separately by domain to ensure that each receives appropriate attention. Assessments are often blue-printed to ensure that all three domains are covered.

Knowledge

Knowledge is the usual starting point. Teachers concentrate a great deal on content and it is important to get this right. What do students need to know? This is not an easy question. Partly, the answer will depend on the formal curriculum from the medical school and the stage the students have reached. What do they already know and what are they interested in? It is important that students find the learning meaningful and can make connections with past learning. It's also good practice to start by asking them what they are hoping for. At first, some may only be interested in 'what's in the exam?' and may need help in seeing the value of any teaching beyond this. It can be helpful to illustrate how the content in psychiatry will be useful to them as doctors when they first qualify, and also the value for a range of specialities.

Having decided what knowledge is needed, the next step is to determine how it should be conveyed. For example, will it be in lecture format, online, or using interactive group methods? Which teaching style you adopt will play a large part in determining how students are able use the knowledge you are imparting. In this context, it is useful to consider Bloom's Taxonomy (Bloom et al., 1956). This taxonomy offers a hierarchical ordering of cognitive skills, from the basic level of remembering, through understanding, and on to more complex activities such as analysis and evaluation. To use knowledge in complex ways, students need opportunities to engage and work with content, and to respond to questioning and assessment that goes beyond knowledge recall.

Skills

The second domain, teaching skill development, requires great care and professionalism on the part of the clinical teacher. Working with patients in psychiatry can be very rewarding for students, but it can also be quite scary and intimidating. The old 'see one, do one, teach one' adage is limited when it comes to the wide range of skills expected of current medical students. Teachers can help by specifying the skills required and by being clear with students what level is expected. The learning environment needs careful management to ensure that it provides appropriate learning opportunities, sometimes for quite large numbers of students. Students value opportunities to observe experienced staff with patients wherever possible. It can also be enormously helpful for them to observe junior staff, who they may perceive as being less difficult to emulate. Junior staff are also reported to be less likely to confuse students by 'cutting corners'. Students also benefit from opportunities to experiment in safe environments (e.g. using role play) before embarking on practice with patients.

One of the most important things with regard to skill development is feedback. Students value constructive feedback, but this is an acquired art for teachers and not as easy as it first appears. It is best to avoid the popular 'sandwich' model of positive-negative-positive. This has become a bit of a cliché and students now wait for the 'but' that comes after the first positive. It can be far more powerful to use an interactive approach, similar to patient centredness or shared decision making. Check with the student how they feel they are doing and help them move towards the next step or goal of their learning. Of course, be prepared to raise serious concerns where necessary, but we have (hopefully) left behind the ritual humiliation reported by previous generations.

Attitudes

By far the most controversial of the three domains is the teaching of attitudes. Some argue that attitudes cannot be taught, and others that they shouldn't be taught. But there are two important ways that attitudes are cultivated in students. The first is implicitly, through role modelling. Students observe the behaviour of clinicians and absorb, by a kind of osmosis, what they believe to be the correct attitudes for them to adopt. Role modelling takes place all the time and cannot be avoided, often presenting students with conflicting messages. Take, for example, inter-professionalism. Students may have been taught that different health professionals are to be treated with equal respect. But on placement they may see something different and, in this example, they may 'learn' to adopt a more hierarchical attitude. So, the best teachers ensure that they 'walk the talk' and that their actions are consistent with their explicit teaching.

There are several well-known psychological experiments that show how people 'see' what they expect to see – made famous in the example of the Invisible Gorilla (Chabris and Simons, 2011). If students are left to make sense of what they see without any form of guidance they may well miss out on huge learning opportunities and leave with a mix of (possibly negative) emotions. But if attitudes are made explicit and students are actively encouraged to discuss and debate the range of views that clinicians can legitimately hold, outlooks can be fostered that are conducive to good medical practice. This requires the clinical teacher to facilitate meaningful and engaging group activities, where all students feel safe to explore, challenge, and modify a range of attitudes, and where students will develop an increasingly complex understanding of the importance of underlying attitudes to clinical practice.

Conclusion

It can be useful to delineate knowledge, skills, and attitudes for teaching purposes but, in the end, all three are inseparable and of equal importance. Psychiatry teachers are among the best placed to offer students a wide range of learning opportunities, involving positive, safe, and challenging experiences in all three domains. A balanced approach, enabling learning across knowledge, skills, and attitudes, is nowhere more important than in mental health.

References

Bloom, B. S., Engelhart, M. D., Furst, E. J., Hill, W. H., and Krathwohl, D. R. (1956). *Taxonomy of Educational Objectives: The Classification of Educational Goals*. Handbook I: Cognitive Domain. New York: David McKay Company.

Chabris, C. and Simons, D. (2011). *The Invisible Gorilla: How Our Intuitions Deceive Us*. Harper Collins.

The Learner

Professor Faith Hill

Teachers tend to focus on what is being taught, but there is much value in putting this aside and focussing on the learner. What do we know about our learners? Medical students are predominantly very bright and arrive at medical school highly motivated. They want to become effective clinicians – to be 'just like you'. But sometimes they seem unprepared, bored, or distracted. What is going wrong?

Student motivation often comes down to basic things like physical comfort. Are your learners cold, or tired, or hungry? It may be that your learners are anxious about their safety, especially in some mental health contexts, and they may need reassurance about this. Or an individual may have emotional issues relating to the subject and be concerned about how it resonates with them or with their family or friends. It is common for students to confront personal issues in the context of psychiatry placements and teachers need to be ready to manage this effectively. Learners also need a sense of belonging and to feel that they are part of the group in which they find themselves. We often assume that students will know each other by the time they are in the third or fourth year, but this is not always the case. They may need time for introductions and establishing 'ground rules' for working together. It can be helpful for the learners to have clear guidance on how, when, and where they will be expected to interact with staff and patients. Do they feel they have a legitimate and valued role within your healthcare setting?

It's also important to address how learning takes place. There are a wide range of education theories that seek to explain how learners learn, and most of these theories offer useful insights for teachers. It is impossible to do justice to them all here, but one theory that is particularly useful in this context is the concept of learning styles.

Four learning styles were originally identified by David Kolb in the 1980s (Kolb, 1984). These are described in Table 1.4.1. The idea is that while each student is unique, they tend to approach learning in one of four ways. The first of these can be described as Innovative Learners, where students prefer to learn through direct experience and reflection. These students seek to understand the reason for what they are asked to do and learn through sensing, feeling, and watching. These learners have been described as imaginative, able to view situations from a range of perspectives, good with people, and influenced by their peers. The second style of learning contrasts sharply with the first. The Analytic Learner prefers to wait and see, lining up the facts in advance of any action. This learning style is good for critiquing information and is common in students who enjoy concepts and models and like to know what the experts think. Analytic Learners are portrayed as thorough and industrious and are comfortable in traditional classrooms and with lectures.

Table 1.4.1 Learning Styles

Learning style	Starting points for learning
Innovative Learner	Student prefers to learn through direct experience and reflection
Analytic Learner	Student prefers to wait and see, getting the facts lined up in advance of any action
Common-Sense Learner	Student is impatient with too much theory or what they may see as 'fuzzy ideas'
Dynamic Learner	Student is primarily interested in self-discovery and prefers to learn by trial and error

The third learning style is sometimes referred to as Common Sense Learning. These learners are impatient with too much theory or what they may see as 'fuzzy ideas'. They seek clear concepts that they can directly apply in practice, and they are good at thinking things through for themselves and at problem solving. They value teachers who let them try things and offer them hands-on experience. The final group of students are Dynamic Learners. These are students who are primarily interested in self-discovery and prefer to learn by trial and error. They like variety and change and are at ease with people. They often learn best by teaching others.

These four styles can be regarded as starting points. While each student may have their preferred style, they will need to apply all these approaches in order to be successful. The student who loves books and libraries will need to develop his or her skills in learning through patient contact. The student who is impatient to get hands-on experience may benefit from more attention to theory and concepts. Part of the teaching role is to offer students a range of learning activities that allow for preferred styles but also encourage flexibility and extension. To achieve this, it can be helpful for teachers to reflect on their own learning style. How do you prefer to learn? And does this determine (or even limit) your approach to teaching? Could you offer a wider range of activities or vary your techniques more?

The concept of learning styles has been developed into the idea of a learning cycle. Teaching that focuses on experiential learning, such as in a problem-based curriculum, is often structured around learning cycles. The idea is that learners need to work through a series of stages in each cycle. The cycle starts with a learning experience – for example, a lecture, observation, patient contact, clinical skills training, role play, media, or film. For learning to take place there must then be opportunity for reflection on the experience, digesting and analysing the content, and making sense of the learning. This is the second stage of learning. The third stage involves learners and teachers introducing new theory that will help the learner grow and develop in response to the experience. This often manifests as 'shall we find out more' or 'let's go away and do some research'. Finally, there is the planning stage, where students consolidate learning and plan ahead for the next learning experience. At this point, one learning cycle is complete but the process is a spiral and the learner now embarks on their next learning experience. The role of the teacher is to facilitate each learning cycle. This cycle is illustrated in Figure 1.4.1.

Figure 1.4.1 The learning spiral

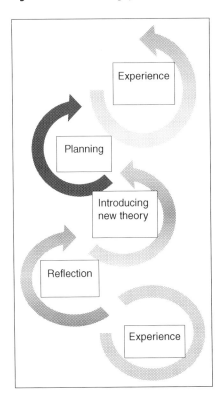

Conclusion

Teachers are often concerned about how to motivate students and sometimes complain that the students are just not interested – they just want to be told what is in the exam. The trick is to shift our gaze away from what we are teaching long enough to focus on who the learners are, what they need, and how they learn.

References

Kolb, D. A. (1984). *Experiential learning: Experience as the source of learning and development.* Englewood Cliffs, NJ: Prentice Hall.

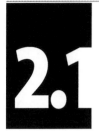

Understanding Curriculum Design

Dr Kenneth Ruddock and Dr Robert Clafferty

Definition

Curriculum design is the overt systematic organisation of an effective, relevant and functional educational programme for the benefit of the students, teachers, and stakeholders involved in a course. It requires clarity of the aims, syllabus, and learning objectives to meet the outcomes regarding knowledge, skills, and attitudes, with careful organisation of educational experiences, learning environment, timetabling and resource distribution. The curriculum should reflect differences in students' learning styles, digital learning options, and local cultural and socio-political environmental factors. A course must be sustainable and embed evaluation and continuous improvement from the outset.

Undergraduate psychiatry curriculum design should specifically reflect our specialty in the broader medical school curriculum and recognise the overlap of psychiatric skills in other areas of the course – for example, psychological aspects of illness in other medical and surgical specialties. A psychiatry course requires more emphasis on biopsychosocial aspects of aetiology and treatment. The potential benefits of a well-designed programme and enjoyable placement include attracting future recruits by showcasing the many benefits of psychiatry (such as flexible working and team support), demonstrating meaningful patient-centred interaction, and offering a chance for our future workforce to develop personal resilience, leadership, and compassionate healthcare skills.

When it is Required

Principles of curriculum design will apply from setting up or reviewing a single learning session to developing an entirely new high-level, strategic, multi-layered course. A static curriculum is a stale curriculum – it requires continual review to ensure it remains relevant and effective, with a process of feedback and quality improvement to inform developments over time (Abrahamson, 1996). A need for review may be prompted if variation is found in benchmarking similar courses or if external agencies such as the General Medical Council (GMC) highlight difficulties. Feedback from students or teachers on a course may identify a sub-optimally performing component, triggering a deeper exploration of the issue.

Curriculum design is a complex process – it is unrealistic to expect to get it perfectly right first time, so incremental change and adaptation is important. Many contextual issues will affect decisions – for example, developing online resources in a short timescale to accommodate the impact of a global pandemic on clinical placement teaching, or the need to design appropriate learning opportunities to support a new entry route for mature students from healthcare backgrounds or postgraduate applicants.

Who is Involved

Curriculum design must reflect the needs of multiple stakeholders, including primarily the students, the teachers (medical and multidisciplinary) and the university (General Medical Council, 2015). Beyond these, the views and requirements of patients, NHS employers and agencies such as the GMC or the Royal College of Psychiatrists (RCPsych) are significant factors. It is important to recognise that the curriculum is influenced by other forces, including local and national politics and public expectations.

To help shape the curriculum, it is essential to have effective leadership; setting up a curriculum review group with appropriate representation can help move the agenda forward. Membership might include students on the course, student society members, faculty staff from academic and clinical backgrounds, administrative staff, educational technology colleagues, and those with responsibility for assessment and examination setting. Opportunities exist for collaboration between medical schools in sharing expertise and resources.

Driving Forces

Medical students need to develop knowledge and clinical skills which reflect the socio-demographic aspects of their future working environments. For example, the changing demographics of UK healthcare suggest future doctors will need increasing skill in managing an elderly population with complex multiple chronic physical and mental health problems (General Medical Council, 2018a). There is an agenda towards matching workforce training to where skills are required most – for example, in rural settings, primary care (Scottish Government, 2019) and, notably, understaffed psychiatric services (Royal College of Psychiatrists, 2019). Doctors' skills in team working, communication, and collaboration have gained prominence, and an awareness of the importance of equality and diversity issues highlights the need to include learning experiences to reduce stigma, support students with mental health problems or physical limitations, remove barriers due to race, gender, sexuality, and gender identification, and support a widening of medical school applicants from a social diversity which represents the general population (General Medical Council, 2017).

Mental health issues have recently been given positive endorsement following high-profile support from the UK royal family and other celebrities. The RCPsych promotes psychiatry with incentives for students to attend conferences and summer schools and compete for prizes, to challenge stigma against psychiatry and to view psychiatry as a positive career choice (Royal College of Psychiatrists, 2019).

Underlying Educational Theory

How Students Learn

The way in which individuals learn has been a topic of debate for many years. Knowledge of learning theory may help develop the pathway from novice rote learning through to higher-order evaluation and mastery of a topic within a curriculum. Increasingly, adult-learner approaches with student-directed elements, access to core and extended material (for students seeking deeper learning) and reflective practice techniques have gained

Table 2.1.1 The FAIR Principles

F	Feedback
A	Activities to engage in active learning
I	Individual interesting opportunities
R	Relevant

prominence, with teachers adapting to often being facilitators rather than providers of didactic information – a 'guide from the side' rather than 'a sage on the stage' (Dacre and Fox, 2000).

Theories of learning for psychiatry which are important when designing a curriculum can at a basic level be demonstrated with reference to the FAIR principles. (Table 2.1.1) These recommend provision of feedback for individual reflection and personal development, inclusion of activities that engage the student in active approaches to learning (i.e. learning by doing rather than passive observation), ensuring learning experiences are individualised for the student and of interest to them, and that they are relevant to the student's needs (Harden and Laidlaw, 2013).

Educational Strategies

Educational strategies are the approach taken to orientate teaching and learning within a curriculum; they must be flexibly adapted over time to reflect the priorities of the educational system and the context of the environment wherein students are learning. A checklist of recognised educational strategies can help when developing or remodelling a curriculum. The SPICES model (Table 2.1.2) is frequently used and refers to six features on a continuum, describing approaches between contemporary and traditional curriculum requirements (Harden, Sowden, and Dunn, 1984). Each curriculum requires a unique blend of 'spices' to function optimally. For some components, learning using a traditional model may have advantages over contemporary approaches, and vice versa.

Contemporary curricula are more focussed on the needs of the students than on those of the medical school. Active engagement of students in curriculum design and learning is encouraged and is demonstrated by increased small-group interactive teaching and personalised learning opportunities – for example, using flexible virtual learning approaches rather than traditional didactic lecture-based approaches.

Rather than an information gathering, rote-learning approach, recent strategies encourage a problem-based learning system; material presented in real-life scenarios links the topic to clinical practice and encourages collaborative team working and peer interaction to solve the problem. In the process, students learn problem-solving techniques, and gain knowledge and the ability to apply it to clinical scenarios (Clark, 2006).

A discipline-based approach is typically used in traditional curricula (Figure 2.1.1, top). A limitation is that students learn a topic (e.g. neuroanatomy) in isolation at one point in the course and may struggle to apply it later, for example when assessing patients with dementia. Integration is an alternative approach, wherein relevant topics are brought together under themes or clinical presentations, for example 'a patient with confusion' (Brauer and Ferguson, 2014).

Table 2.1.2 The SPICES model

S	Student centred
P	Problem based
I	Integrated
C	Community based
E	Elective and core
S	Systematic

Teaching students in hospital-based settings alone does not reflect the high number of students who identify community-based specialties (including many branches of Psychiatry) and General Practice as their career aspiration. Offering learning opportunities outside of hospital settings gives students experience of the health needs of local communities and the flow and context of care in community settings.

Systematic approaches are recommended to ensure students see the breadth of clinical scenarios and do not graduate with gaps in their knowledge. Relying on opportunistic learning on placements or apprenticeship approaches can give patchy experience. Methods to help overcome such issues include simulation, clinical skills sessions, clinical logbooks, and portfolios, as well as setting clear learning outcomes and ensuring learning objectives are aligned to cover them.

Curriculum Models

The fundamental structure and model of the overarching curriculum relies on the basic underlying framework. Several varieties exist, having gained and lost favour over time (Papa and Harasym, 1999); usually there will be elements of different types evident in a contemporary course, and it is important to note that one size does not fit all. Themes such as apprenticeship, discipline/system, and problem-based methods may be present in parts of the course. Recent moves towards outcome-based education have gained prominence (Ross, Hauer and Melle, 2018). Fundamental arrangements regarding pre-clinical/clinical separation compared to an integrated model and decisions regarding inclusion of elective and special study modules (SSMs) to individualise a student experience must be considered. Psychiatry might be taught within horizontal or modular blocks, though it and related themes typically have a place in vertical and spirally arranged curricula models (Figure 2.1.1, bottom).

RCPsych recommends that psychiatry should feature throughout the undergraduate curriculum and be better integrated with basic sciences and physical health rather than restricted to a single block in the final years of medical school, as is often the case (Royal College of Psychiatrists, 2019). Earlier exposure to psychiatry may increase students' likelihood of choosing psychiatry as a career and make them less likely to develop stigmatising attitudes towards mental illness (Royal College of Psychiatrists, 2019).

The GMC recommends integrating medical school curricula with clinical exposure from an early stage, and creating options for students to choose areas of study in which they are interested (General Medical Council, 2015).

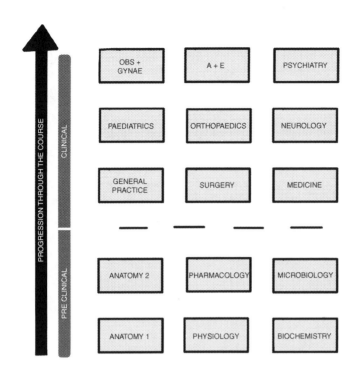

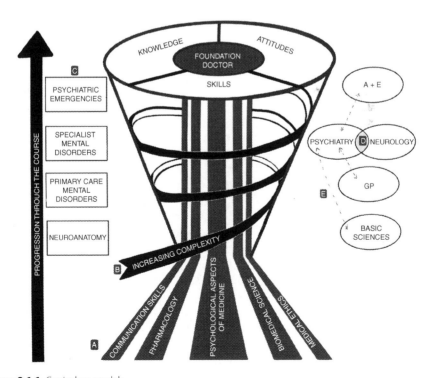

Figure 2.1.1 Curriculum models

Top: Traditional curriculum with pre-clinical/clinical modular design

Bottom: Contemporary curriculum with A) Vertical themes, B) Spiral Iterative learning opportunities, C) Integration via themed placements, D) Horizontal module linking and E) Vertical module linking

One organisational method is to use a 'spiral curriculum' framework incorporating both horizontal and vertical themes. The spiral curriculum involves revisiting the same educational topics over the course of a student's education with increasing levels of complexity, whilst achieving progressively deeper knowledge (Harden, 1999).

Integration of learning can take place either vertically – with common themes (e.g. pharmacology and therapeutics) running across the years, spanning basic sciences and clinical phases (e.g. neuroanatomy with clinical psychiatry) – or horizontally, where there is integration between different clinical presentations (e.g. fatigue), subject areas (e.g. pathology and physiology), or medical specialties (e.g. Paediatrics with Child and Adolescent Mental Health) (Brauer and Ferguson, 2014; Hays, 2013). Integration helps ensure students appreciate that mental illness is a fundamental aspect of many presentations of disease, and research suggests this may normalise approaches to mental health and improve general attitudes towards psychiatry (Royal College of Psychiatrists, 2019).

Determining the Course Content

Defining Learning Aims, Objectives and Outcomes

The terms 'learning aims', 'learning objectives', and 'learning outcomes' are confusingly similar and are often used interchangeably; however, they have distinct meanings within medical education.

A learning aim is a concise description of the overall goal of a teaching programme or session. A statement of aims should reflect the values, principles, and requirements from stakeholders and the essence of clinical skills required to succeed in the course. It should guide students and teachers alike as to what is expected of them when they participate in the programme.

A learning objective is a brief description of how learning aims are going to be fulfilled, usually written from the perspective of the teacher, and may include what teaching methods will be used, what students will be doing, and what the students are expected to learn. This may cover knowledge, skills, and attitudes. Learning objectives should be strategically coordinated to avoid omission or duplication in other parts of the course.

An intended learning outcome focuses on what students will be doing and offers a concise statement of how learners will demonstrate evidence to confirm they have achieved a learning objective. Learning outcomes offer standardisation between courses and may be guided by external requirements such as the GMC Licensing Exam. They should be 'SMART': that is, specific, measurable, appropriate, realistic, and time bound. Typically, they are recorded in the future tense and state what students should be able to do after a teaching session. They may range in increasing sophistication from novice to expert in a hierarchy of complexity – based upon Bloom's taxonomy – and should include action verbs. Clearly written learning outcomes will guide educators in designing constructively aligned course content, help students identify what they are required to learn, and provide a clear basis for assessment.

Examples of a learning aim, a learning objective, and learning outcomes for a course are provided in Table 2.1.3. A learning outcome is provided for each level of Bloom's revised taxonomy (Anderson, Krathwohl, and Bloom, 2001).

Table 2.1.3 Exemplar learning aim, learning objective, and learning outcomes

Learning aim	To gain experience in the assessment, diagnosis, and management of depression
Learning objective	To recognise the symptoms of depression and the role of antidepressant prescription in the biopsychosocial management of patients by attending a multidisciplinary affective disorder assessment clinic
Learning outcomes	By the of this course the student should be able to:
- Remember:	List the ICD-11 core symptoms of depression
- Understand:	Describe the monoamine hypothesis of depression
- Apply:	Explain antidepressant drug treatment options to a patient
- Analyse:	Develop a management plan for a patient presenting with low mood
- Evaluate:	Compare SIGN and NICE guidelines for antidepressant drug treatment options
- Create:	Design a new clinical algorithm to support evidence-based choice of antidepressants in your service

Determining the Core Content

In developing a psychiatry curriculum, several external standards must be taken into consideration, both in benchmarking between similar educational establishments and in adhering to national agency guidelines. In the United Kingdom these include the GMC's 'Outcomes for Graduates' recommendations and the model curriculum from the RCPsych. Basing the course on a recognised syllabus is a good starting point. A helpful approach may be to complete an appraisal of what is already in an existing curriculum using a curriculum mapping process.

Syllabus Review

The syllabus is a list of the taught content of a course. It will reflect the professional regulators' expectations with typical topics, including basic science, clinical descriptions of psychiatric conditions, biopsychosocial formulation, multidisciplinary management, differentiation of normal life events from mental illness, awareness of how mental health services are structured, mental health legislation, and risk assessment and management. It might be recorded in a bespoke study guide or online resource developed for the course, or be available in a carefully chosen aligned course textbook.

Curriculum Mapping

Curriculum mapping involves reviewing the course content to ensure that learning outcomes are appropriately covered within educational sessions and there are no unintentional omissions or duplications of learning objectives (Al-Eyd et al., 2018). Mapping offers a strategic blueprint overview of the whole course and can be particularly helpful in reviewing and planning developments in the curriculum and in giving clear direction to staff charged with the task of providing educational experiences aligned to the required learning outcomes (Harden, 2001).

GMC Outcomes for Graduates

The GMC divides outcomes into three key domains: professional values and behaviours, professional skills, and professional knowledge (General Medical Council, 2018a). Many of the GMC's outcomes are relevant to mental health care and can be addressed during the psychiatry specialty block or at other stages throughout the course.

Professional values and behaviours are underpinned by the key principle that newly qualified doctors 'must make the care of their patients their first concern, applying their knowledge and skills in a competent, ethical and professional manner and taking responsibility for their own actions in complex and uncertain situations' (General Medical Council, 2018a, p. 7).

Professional skills take account of communication, interpersonal skills, diagnosis, and medical management. Key skills relevant to psychiatry include history-taking (particularly from patients with communication difficulties or those with an insight-impairing illness), performing a mental and cognitive state examination, and establishing whether a patient is a risk to themselves or others.

Professional knowledge covers principles of biomedical science, social sciences, and illness. Doctors should be able to describe the spectrum of normal human behaviour, explain the relationship between psychological and medical conditions, and explain how psychological factors may impact treatment outcomes.

Being aware of the explicit standards set by the GMC for medical graduates is in line with the outcome-based education model. This requires the curriculum to focus on a clear set of essential standards that students must be able to demonstrate they 'know and are capable of' on completion of the course (Harden, 2007). Working backwards from this, curriculum planners can set learning outcomes, arrange learning objectives, and reflect the requirements in the aims of their course.

RCPsych Curriculum

The RCPsych 'Core Curriculum in Psychiatry' (Royal College of Psychiatrists, 2017), provides a detailed blueprint for what should be included in undergraduate psychiatry training. Specific content and level of depth is left at the discretion of medical schools. The overall aim of the curriculum is for newly qualified doctors to 'be able to recognise, assess and diagnose mental illness, manage psychiatric emergencies effectively, and know when to refer to seniors and to psychiatric specialists'.

The curriculum is based upon the GMC's 'Outcomes for Graduates (Tomorrow's Doctors)' document from 2015, with learning outcomes presented across three overarching themes: the doctor as a scholar and scientist, the doctor as a practitioner, the doctor as a professional.

'The doctor as a scholar and scientist' theme covers knowledge of common psychiatric disorders; pharmacological, physical, social, and psychological therapies; and principles of psychiatric formulation. Within 'the doctor as a practitioner' theme, the curriculum advises that students should be able to take a full psychiatric history, conduct a mental state examination, assess capacity, and safely prescribe psychopharmacological treatments.

Finally, 'the doctor as a professional' theme states that students should behave according to ethical and legal principles, recognise the importance of developing a therapeutic relationship, understand the role of the multidisciplinary team, and recognise the importance of maintaining one's own mental health and well-being. The RCPsych curriculum also includes appendices which detail specific topics which should be covered.

Organising Specific Course Components

Arranging Learning Experiences

There are a wide range of options to consider when organising educational experiences, the choice of which will be based on various factors, including university facilities, clinical placement availability, access to technology, faculty size, and student numbers. There is little evidence to suggest that one approach is better than another (Grant, 2014); however, it is important to align learning appropriately- for example, communication skills may be more suitably learnt in a small interactive simulation session rather than in a large group lecture. It is essential to ensure there is a balance between online and in-person teaching experience.

Suggested approaches to teaching include the provision of physical or online course textbooks, lectures (useful for teaching fundamental sciences and essential knowledge to large numbers simultaneously, either in traditional delivery or supported by flipped classroom techniques), and small group tutorials/workshops (useful when student interaction is required- for example, during problem or case-based learning or role-play/simulation sessions; Grant, 2014). Other methods include online delivery; pre-recorded lectures or live online tutorials are useful, particularly when students are accommodated in peripheral sites and unable to return to the university for teaching. Some components may be supported via a Virtual Learning Environment (VLE); digital modules can support student learning where there is access to appropriate software and technological support. Traditional bedside/patient-focussed teaching remains a fundamental requirement in psychiatry, to target skills related to history-taking or eliciting psychopathology; these can be supplemented by reflective learning (e.g. Balint groups) and with peer-assisted approaches such as study guides, checklist practice, and supported study groups.

When organising a clinical placement there are several practical factors to consider. It is helpful to provide a timetable for teaching in advance and to ensure the student is welcomed into the team. Providing an induction with tour of facilities, giving information on safety measures in clinical environments, and telling them who to contact if they experience any difficulties will help settle students. It is also helpful to consider issues of travel between community sites and accommodation support. It may be possible to arrange additional specialist sessions for students who are particularly interested in a subspecialty of psychiatry if these are not offered elsewhere in the placement.

Developing Resources

The resources required will depend on which teaching approaches are being taken and may include reading lists, lecture slides (and transcripts if lectures are pre-recorded), facilitator guides (e.g. for communication skills workshops or simulation sessions), study guides/ workbooks, clinical logbooks, advance preparation for flipped classroom sessions, multimedia resources (videos or podcast recordings), formative assessment, and topic quizzes. If these resources are centralised the course material can be standardised, which will allow consistency if multiple teachers provide training sessions over the course of an academic year.

To support sustainability, there may be more reliance on paperless resources, with educational materials being accessible from virtual learning platforms. In the United Kingdom, the MyPsych App is utilised by several medical schools; this provides electronic resources for students, including links to guidelines and educational videos (McKee et al., 2017).

When designing a new curriculum for psychiatry, much work may be required at the outset to develop course materials to cover all learning outcomes. This is an opportunity to divide the workload and to seek assistance from academic and clinical colleagues. Psychiatry trainees may have an interest in medical education and can assist in the development of teaching materials. Students themselves may play a key role in developing resources. There may be opportunities to collaborate and share resources with other medical schools. Once resources have been developed, it is necessary to have a system to review content to ensure it remains up to date.

Developing Teachers

A successful course relies on a cohort of knowledgeable and enthusiastic educators. These can be drawn from a wide range of backgrounds and grades, including academic staff, consultants, staff grade/specialty doctors, doctors in training, and non-medical colleagues, such as nurses and psychologists. Though clinical staff may find it challenging to ring-fence time for teaching, the GMC advises that all doctors 'should be prepared to contribute to teaching and training doctors and students' (General Medical Council, 2018b, p. 14), and evidence of teaching activity is useful for appraisal and revalidation purposes (General Medical Council, 2009). Junior doctors can be recruited as 'near-peer' educators or mentors for medical students during clinical placements. Some teachers may be interested in becoming involved in developing or updating the curriculum, bringing new insights and experiences from their own practice.

Supporting educators with continuing professional development events can equip them with the knowledge and skills to be high-quality teachers or examiners (General Medical Council, 2009). Teaching observations provide an opportunity for constructive feedback regarding teaching methods and delivery.

Student Welfare

In recent years there has been increased focus on student welfare, with medical schools improving resources and facilities embedded within the curriculum to better meet the needs of their students (British Medical Association, 2019). Medical students are at increased risk of stress and burnout, as well as psychiatric illnesses such as depression, anxiety, eating disorders, and substance-use disorders (General Medical Council, 2013). It is well established that medical students and doctors are prone to neglect their own physical and mental health (Hooper, Meakin, and Jones, 2005).

Student welfare and well-being can be considered as a vertical theme which is relevant throughout all stages of the undergraduate curriculum. The GMC states that newly qualified doctors 'must demonstrate awareness of the need to self-monitor, self-care and seek appropriate advice and support' as well as 'manage the personal and emotional challenges of coping with work and workload … [and] develop a range of coping strategies' (General Medical Council, 2018a, p. 10).

Psychiatrists are well placed to identify when students may be experiencing difficulties. Issues may not arise until psychiatry placements when students are confronted with challenging topics they may have had experience of personally or through family or friends. Such students may require tailored support during their placement or input from the student welfare service.

Assessment

Student Examination

Students' self-reported drive to study is directly influenced by the content of course exams: 'assessment drives learning' (Wood, 2009; Wormald et al., 2009). A carefully designed curriculum should be constructively aligned, with assessment matched to course content and intended learning outcomes (Biggs, 1996).

The choice of assessment will depend on which aspects of the curriculum – knowledge, skills, or attitudes – are being assessed. Multiple-choice questions, short answer questions, and extended matching items are useful for assessing knowledge, whereas objective structured clinical examination (OSCE) or direct observation clinical examination stations assess clinical skills such as history-taking and mental state examination (Epstein, 2007). Attitudes can be more difficult to assess; these may be included within an OSCE station – in the form of a global examiner rating – or can be considered within a case report reflective log (Shumway and Harden, 2003). Professionalism assessment may be based upon student attendance, conduct, and level of engagement during a clinical placement.

Students' assessment performance provides a measure of whether the curriculum and educational experiences meet their learning needs (Grant, 2014). Areas of weakness within assessment may highlight deficits in course content and guide future changes to the curriculum.

Course Evaluation

Evaluation is an essential component of the education process. It can be used to ensure teaching is meeting students' learning needs, identify areas of good practice, or indicate where there are improvement needs for individual teachers or any other component of the curriculum (Morrison, 2003). Regular cycles of evaluation and quality improvement should take place.

Feedback should be gathered from students, teachers, and course organisers and may be in person or online. It is useful to collect a mixture of qualitative and quantitative feedback. Students should be made aware of the outcomes of the evaluation process and any resulting action that has been taken. This helps students to see that their opinions are valued and keeps them engaged in the feedback process (Morrison, 2003).

Conclusion

Curriculum design is an essential, challenging, yet rewarding aspect of undergraduate medical education. It requires knowledge of underlying education theory and principles, collaboration from various interested parties, administrative support, energy, drive, and commitment. Recognising how psychiatry fits into an overall educational system helps to highlight its importance as a core aspect of medical school learning. Taking time to plan effective learning, be it for a whole course or a single session, is a rewarding experience – your students and their future patients will thank you for it.

References

Abrahamson S. (1996). *Essays on Medical Education*. University Press of America.

Al-Eyd, G., Achike, F., Agarwal, M., et al. (2018). Curriculum mapping as a tool to facilitate curriculum development: A new School of Medicine experience. *BMC Medical Education*, **18** (1): 185.

Anderson, L., Krathwohl, D., and Bloom, B. (2001). *A Taxonomy For Learning, Teaching, And Assessing*. New York: Longman.

Biggs, J. (1996). Enhancing teaching through constructive alignment. *Higher Education*, **32**, 347–64.

Brauer, D. and Ferguson, K. (2014). The integrated curriculum in medical education: AMEE Guide No. 96. *Medical Teacher*, **37** (4): 312–22.

British Medical Association. (2019). Mental health and wellbeing in the medical profession: report 2019. (Online) Available at: www.bma.org.uk/media/1361/bma-mental-health-and-wellbeing-medical-profession-research-summary-oct-2019.pdf (accessed 5 December 2020).

Clark, C. E. (2006). Problem-based learning: How do the outcomes compare with traditional teaching? *British Journal of General Practice*, **56** (530): 722–3.

Dacre, J. E. and Fox, R. A. (2000). How should we be teaching our undergraduates? *Annals of the Rheumatic Diseases*, **59** (9): 662–7.

Epstein, R. (2007). Assessment in medical education. *New England Journal of Medicine*, **356** (4): 387–96.

General Medical Council. (2009). Developing teachers and trainers in undergraduate medical education. (Online) Available at: www.gmc-uk.org/-/media/documents/Developing_teachers_and_trainers_in_undergraduate_medical_education___

guidance_0815.pdf_56440721.pdf (accessed 28 November 2020).

General Medical Council. (2013). Supporting medical students with mental health conditions. (Online) Available at: www.gmc-uk.org/-/media/documents/Supporting_students_with_mental_health_conditions_0816.pdf_53047904.pdf (accessed 30 November 2020).

General Medical Council. (2015). Promoting excellence: Standards for medical education and training. (Online) Available at: www.gmc-uk.org/-/media/documents/promoting-excellence-standards-for-medical-education-and-training-0715_pdf-61939165.pdf (accessed 28 November 2020).

General Medical Council. (2017). Promoting excellence – equality and diversity considerations. (Online) Available at: www.gmc-uk.org/education/standards-guidance-and-curricula/guidance/promoting-excellence-equality-and-diversity-considerations (accessed 5 December 2020).

General Medical Council. (2018a). Outcomes for graduates. (Online) Available at: www.gmc-uk.org/-/media/documents/outcomes-for-graduates-2020_pdf-84622587.pdf (accessed 28 November 2020).

General Medical Council. (2018b). Good medical practice. (Online) Available at: www.gmc-uk.org/ethical-guidance/ethical-guidance-for-doctors/good-medical-practice (accessed 28 November 2020).

Grant, J. (2014). Principles of curriculum design. In T. Swanwick, ed., *Understanding medical education: Evidence, theory and practice*, 2nd ed. Wiley Blackwell. https://doi.org/10.1002/9781118472361.ch3.

Harden, R. M. (1999). What is a spiral curriculum? *Medical Teacher*, **21** (2): 141–3.

Harden, R. M. (2001). AMEE Guide No. 21: Curriculum mapping: A tool for transparent and authentic teaching and learning. *Medical Teacher*, **23** (2): 123–37.

Harden, R. M. (2007). Outcome-based education: The future is today. *Medical Teacher*, **29**, 625–9.

Harden, R. M. and Laidlaw, J. M. (2013). Be FAIR to students: four principles that lead to more effective learning. *Medical Teacher*, **35** (1): 27–31.

Harden, R. M., Sowden, S. and Dunn, W. R. (1984). Educational strategies in curriculum development: The SPICES model. *Medical Education*, **18** (4): 284–97.

Hays, H. (2013). Integration in medical education: What do we mean? *Education for Primary Care*, **24**, 151–2.

Hooper, C., Meakin, R., and Jones, M. (2005). Where students go when they are ill: How medical students access health care. *Medical Education*, **9** (6): 588–593.

McKee, T., Penades, N., Wolfe, M., and Ogston, N. (2017). MyPsych – a psychiatry placement app for medical students. (Poster). *Scottish Medical Education Conference*. Edinburgh, May 2017. Available at: www.researchgate .net/publication/311101431_MyPsych_-_a_ psychiatry_placement_app_for_medical_ students (accessed 5 December 2020).

Morrison, J. (2003). ABC of learning and teaching in medicine: Evaluation. *British Medical Journal*, **326** (7385): 385–7.

Papa, F. and Harasym, P. (1999). Medical curriculum reform in North America 1765 to the present: a cognitive perspective. *Academic Medicine*, **74**, 154–64.

Ross, S., Hauer, K., and Melle, E. (2018). Outcomes are what matter: Competency-based medical education gets us to our goal. *MedEd Publish* (7)2, 17.

Royal College of Psychiatrists. (2017). Core curriculum in psychiatry. (Online) Available at: www.rcpsych.ac.uk/docs/default-source/ training/training/undergraduate-curriculum-2017—2021-revision—academic-faculty.pdf? sfvrsn=bc103cb6_2 (accessed 28 November 2020).

Royal College of Psychiatrists. (2019). Choose psychiatry: Guidance for medical schools. (Online) Available at: www.rcpsych.ac.uk/ docs/default-source/become-a-psychiatrist/ guidance-for-medical-schools-pdf.pdf?sfvrsn= 20f46cae_2 (accessed 5 December 2020).

Scottish Government. (2019). Undergraduate medical education in Scotland: Enabling more general practice based teaching – final report. (Online) Available at: www.gov.scot/ publications/undergraduate-medical-education-scotland-enabling-more-general-practice-based-teaching/ (accessed 5 December 2020).

Shumway, J. M. and Harden, R. M. (2003). AMEE Guide No. 25: The assessment of learning outcomes for the competent and reflective physician. *Medical Teacher*, **25** (6): 569–84.

Wood, T. (2009). Assessment not only drives learning, it may also help learning. *Medical Education*, **43** (1): 5–6.

Wormald, B., Schoeman, S., Somasunderam, A., and Penn, M. (2009). Assessment drives learning: An unavoidable truth? *Anatomical Sciences Education*, **2** (5): 199–204.

Preclinical Versus Clinical Years

Dr Neelom Sharma

Psychological Aspects of Medicine

What should we teach medical students about mental health in the preclinical years? Traditionally, this has been virtually nothing (Karim, 2009), and it is not unusual for students starting their clinical years to be unaware of the differences between psychiatrists and psychologists, for example.

Recent years have seen changes; the first 'Tomorrow's Doctors' document (GMC, 1993) did not make reference to psychiatry or psychology, with only brief mention of mental health: 'communicating with people with mental illness, including cases where patients have special difficulties in sharing how they feel and think with doctors' (p. 13).

As shown in Table 2.2.1, the 2009 Tomorrow's Doctors publication (GMC, 2009) marked a turning point, with psychological principles moving to a clear, prominent role in overarching outcomes for medical graduates.

Although Outcomes for Graduates (GMC, 2018) updates these outcomes further, they are broadly similar to those from 2009. Some lend themselves better to early undergraduate years than others. For example, outcome (b) may be considered primarily sociological, so might be best delivered in the early years by a combination of sociologists and clinicians (as we have done in Edinburgh), while (d) might be best delivered by mental health experts within horizontal modules (such as puerperal psychiatric disorders within an Obstetrics module, or depression in chronic illness within a Diabetes module). Others, such as (g), will be core learning outcomes within the Psychiatry module.

Methods of teaching have changed dramatically in the last twenty years (Walsh, 2013), and different medical schools have adapted these at different speeds, with different emphases. Some medical schools have adopted a problem-based learning (PBL) approach in radical ways (Walsh, 2013); others have kept more traditional formats. The emphasis on deep learning marks a change from the 'rote learning' model which preceded it. The flipped classroom has evolved in the internet age (Walsh, 2013), with an enforced and sudden acceleration in implementation with the COVID-19 pandemic.

Most medical schools have adopted PBL to varying degrees in the preclinical years (Walsh, 2013), and psychiatrists co-authoring PBL cases is an ideal way of ensuring many GMC-enshrined outcomes are covered meaningfully. The psychiatrist has an additional role here; as a medical practitioner who is relatively 'deskilled' in acute medical work, the level at which a PBL case is 'pitched' to students in Years 1–2 is more likely to be appropriate to their stage of learning. When I co-authored PBL cases in Edinburgh in 2011–14, it was apparent that several of the pre-existing PBL cases were highly complex 'walk throughs' of a patient journey with a specific illness (e.g. MS or rheumatoid arthritis), written brilliantly by experts

Table 2.2.1 Tomorrow's Doctors, Learning Outcomes, Psychological Aspects of Medicine (GMC, 2009)

Apply psychological principles, method and knowledge to medical practice.
(a) Explain normal human behaviour at an individual level.
(b) Discuss psychological concepts of health, illness and disease.
(c) Apply theoretical frameworks of psychology to explain the varied responses of individuals, groups and societies to disease.
(d) Explain psychological factors that contribute to illness, the course of the disease and the success of treatment.
(e) Discuss psychological aspects of behavioural change and treatment compliance.
(f) Discuss adaptation to major life changes, such as bereavement; comparing and contrasting the abnormal adjustments that might occur in these situations.
(g) Identify appropriate strategies for managing patients with dependence issues and other demonstrations of self harm (GMC, 2009, p. 15).

in the field, but pitched at a level which preclinical students could never be expected to function at. PBL is a great opportunity to meaningfully present many important psychological concepts to preclinical and clinical-years students in a way which ensures that **all** students have covered the content (i.e. mapped), and it is easily assessed. This approach encourages student participation and deep learning.

Lectures may still have a limited role in introducing concepts to students (and this may be particularly true in an age of online lectures, where tools such as electronic polling and presentation of interactive content such as videos and virtual whiteboards can be used). An example may be an Introduction to Psychiatry within Years 1 or 2.

We have found that providing a 'bridge' between preclinical and clinical years is useful. Our bridge in the last few years has been to pair up with Ethicists to deliver a whole-year teaching day on Ethics and Psychological Aspects of Medicine in the 1st semester of the first Clinical Year.

Introductory lectures open the day, before small tutorial groups discuss theoretical but challenging cases. These cover issues such as overdose, treatment refusal, mental health and incapacity legislation, domestic abuse, assisted dying, and the legal framework around medicine. Small-group discussion feels important for this 'bridge'; while we are expecting graduates to possess these competencies at the end of medical school, exploring them in a safe, supportive setting when they start their clinical years is nurturing.

These foundations are built on in their horizontal modules (ostensibly 'medical' ones such as Respiratory or Gastrointestinal medicine), but also in a short Psychiatry course which focuses on how to do a mental state examination and the language used, as well as cognitive assessments. A key function of this course is – for the first time in the curriculum – to meet psychiatric patients in the supported settings of tutorial groups, before independently seeing patients in the second clinical year, where the main Psychiatry module sits.

Stigma

Considerable research shows that medical students starting medical school display similar levels of stigma towards mental illness as the general population, as one might expect (Cutler, 2009).

By the time students graduate, their attitudes have hardened; they are significantly more stigmatising of mental illness (Cutler, 2009). This is unfortunate and will be detrimental to patient care, as well as potentially resulting in doctors being less likely to seek treatment for mental disorders themselves (Thornicroft, 2016). Would adding more preclinical teaching on mental disorders help to minimise or reverse this phenomenon? A recent project by University of Edinburgh medical students robustly demonstrated that Year 1 students carried the same level of stigma as Year 6 students (Kumar and Sharma, 2019), suggesting that the interventions outlined above may have arrested the hardening of attitudes which typically occurs. One might argue that we have therefore done half the job, and that greater efforts are needed to reduce stigmatisation of mental disorders among our future doctors.

Preclinical Input from People with Lived Experience

Gordon Johnston

The introduction of lived experience input here can also assist in developing an early understanding of the psychological aspects of medicine. Hearing lived experience stories and experiences directly can enable students to develop a sense of the patient as a person, rather than simply a combination of symptoms and diagnoses.

Students can also be encouraged to develop the relationship-based approach that will be necessary in all aspects of medicine, enhancing their listening skills and beginning to understand how mental illness can affect life in a manner beyond simple symptomology. Students can also be introduced to concepts of self-management in mental illness and the use of recovery-based approaches, as well as the concept of working in partnership with a patient to achieve good outcomes.

Discussions on challenging stigma around mental health can also be enhanced by the presence of people with lived experience. Understanding of stigma and discrimination from the perspective of those facing it can be much deeper than a purely theoretical consideration can allow.

Self-Awareness and Avoiding Burnout

In medicine it is well-recognised that our jobs affect us profoundly (West, 2016). It is clear that the current generation of medical students are much more aware of their internal worlds than those that have gone before, and that there is greater awareness of the need to avoid burnout (West, 2016). Reflective practice, perhaps in the form of Balint Groups or similar, provides non-judgemental spaces in which students can discuss cases which have challenged them and their emotional responses to them (Muench, 2018). This is something which we have introduced to all students in their first clinical year (as well as to Foundation Year 2 students in Psychiatry and other professional groups), and it has received positive feedback. Again, providing this experience in the first clinical year, during a GP module, feels like an effective way of both bridging the preclinical and clinical years and of teaching important, career-sustaining skills and attitudes to students. This training is delivered by higher trainees experienced in Balint techniques, supervised by the Psychotherapy department. While such extensive resources may not be universally available, it should be possible for Balint Groups to be delivered to students in their undergraduate years in many medical schools. Measuring longitudinal outcomes from such work is challenging.

Challenges to Integration Across the Curriculum

Having been involved in this area for many years, a key challenge has been integration into many different courses. Inevitably, some Module and Year Organisers are more receptive to Psychological and Psychiatric content being part of their module than others. Some courses lend themselves to integration, such as Sociology and Neuroscience in preclinical years, Obstetrics or A&E in clinical years, so these have been our focus.

Labyrinthine, densely packed curricula present further challenges: content can get 'lost' in redesigns. While keeping abreast of curriculum changes is advisable, the range of meetings and number of modules, year and theme organisers make this logistically challenging.

Mapping curriculum content to assessment is a further obstacle. In preclinical years, the primary assessment formats are essay questions and multiple-choice questions (MCQs). Contributing to both can be useful and satisfying, though the key is to ensure that the content being assessed clearly maps to the delivered content. Students (very reasonably) complain if content of a course which is peripheral to the 'main' course they are studying is assessed at all, let alone if content relating to the assessment was not explicitly delivered. Moving into clinical years, OSCEs (objective structured clinical examinations) often predominate. Delivering and assessing OSCEs in the first clinical year is another useful bridge – an ostensibly 'medical' presentation with a psychological basis (such as panic attacks presenting to A&E or Respiratory Medicine) have been stations we have usefully delivered for many years.

Summary

Psychiatry can and should be taught across the entire medical curriculum. While this can present challenges, a wide range of teaching and assessment techniques can be used to help future doctors to be psychologically aware, resilient, empathic practitioners.

References

Cutler, J., Harding, K. J., Mozian, S. A. et al. (2009). Discrediting the notion, 'working with "crazies" will make you "crazy".' Addressing stigma and enhancing empathy in medical student education. *Advances in Health Sciences Education*, **14** (4): 487–502.

GMC. (1993). *Tomorrow's Doctors: Recommendations on Undergraduate Medical Education*. London: General Medical Council.

GMC. (2009). *Tomorrow's Doctors – Updated Version*. London: General Medical Council.

GMC. (2018). *Outcomes for Graduates*. [Online] Available at: www.gmc-uk.org/-/media/ documents/outcomes-for-graduates-a4-6_pdf-78952372.pdf (accessed 7th September 2020).

Karim, K., Edwards, R., Dogra, N., et al. (2009). A survey of the teaching and assessment of undergraduate psychiatry in the medical schools of the United Kingdom and Ireland. *Medical Teacher*, **32** (11): 1024–9.

Kumar, S. and Sharma, N. (2019). *Undergraduate Teaching in Psychological Aspects of Medicine: A Literature Review, Survey and Action Plan*. London: Royal College of Psychiatrists Faculty of Medical Education.

Muench, J. (2018). Balint work and the creation of medical knowledge. *International Journal of Psychiatry in Medicine*, **53** (1–2): 15–23.

Thornicroft, G., Mehta, N., Clement, S. et al. (2016). Evidence for effective interventions to reduce mental-health-related stigma and discrimination. *The Lancet*, **387** (10023): 1123–32.

Walsh, K. (ed.) (2013). *Oxford Textbook of Medical Education*. 1st ed. Oxford: Oxford University Press.

West, C., Dyrbye, L. N., Erwin, P. J., and Shanafelt, T. D. (2016). Interventions to prevent and reduce physician burnout: A systematic review and meta-analysis. *The Lancet*, **388** (10057): 2272–81.

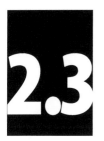

Patients as Educators in Psychiatry: The Ethical and Educational Case

Simon Rose, Alexa Sidwell, and Professor Subodh Dave

William Osler's oft-quoted advice 'To study the phenomena of disease without books is to sail an uncharted sea, while to study books without patients is not to go to sea at all' captures the importance of learning medicine from patients (Osler, 1901). While learning in the clinical setting may be the cornerstone of medical education, service pressures often lead to clinical education taking a backseat to clinical practice.

The introduction of standardised patients (see Chapter 4.5: Simulation) was a step towards maintaining experiential learning in the clinical setting (Barrows, 1993). While standardised patients (which includes both simulated and real patients) offer consistency (Cleland, 2009), there is an inherent paradox in teaching empathy using simulation, especially when an observer is commenting on one's empathic skills. Direct patient feedback can help students understand the way their communication style is experienced by the patient. Such patient feedback is important in facilitating the *experience* of empathy in contrast to enacting empathy – the latter being an attribute sometimes seen in novice trainees in psychiatry.

Why Involve Patients (and Carers) in Training

Policy Case

Over the last two decades, there has been a significant shift in policy for the inclusion of service users in the organisation, planning, and delivery of services (Department of Health, 2001; Mental Health and Social Exclusion, 2004) and also for higher education institutions to involve service users in health professionals' training (Department of Health, 1999).

Consequently, there has been considerable growth in the development of educational programmes that involve service users in their delivery, along with service users providing feedback on student's skills in order to improve their clinical consultation skills (Lai et al., 2020). More recently, the Five Year Forward View for Mental Health, published in 2016 states: 'There should be an even greater emphasis put on peoples' experience and how experts-by-experience be seen as real assets to design and develop services' (p. 18). This push for patient involvement in design of services also makes a strong case for similar partnerships in psychiatric education (Tew et al., 2004).

Ethical Case

The principle of 'doing *with*' rather than 'doing *to*' is well established in relation to clinical practice, with the advent of person-centred care and this principle is now being extended to teaching and training (RCPsych College Report CR215). Translating this ethical principle to action should lead to the involvement of people with lived experience in the design and delivery of teaching and, indeed, of assessment. The principle of co-production demonstrates that respect for patients is egalitarian and challenges stigma (RCPsych College Report CR204; NCCMH, 2019).

Educational Case

Irrespective of the ethics- or values-based case, it is vital that patient involvement in teaching is predicated on its educational impact. Learning from patients with lived experience enables learning to take place within the context of a person's subjective and cultural narrative, providing a deeper meaning to the learning experience. This makes the learning more memorable and reproducible (Jha, 2009b; RCPsych College Report CR215).

Moreover, students get to hear the first-hand account of the patient journey, which provides a different and, crucially, independent perspective to that of healthcare providers. Receiving learning through a collaborative, co-produced educational session serves as a model for a collaborative, co-produced approach in clinical practice. While patient involvement in training improves knowledge and understanding of the patient perspective and helps develop patient-centric attitudes, it also helps foster therapeutic relationship-building skills and advanced communication skills relevant to psychiatric practice (Byren et al., 2013; Tew et al., 2004). This is particularly important given worries about the erosion of empathy in medical students over the course of their medical education (Hojat, 2009). Finally, the involvement of patients in meaningful educational activity enables students to see recovery in action.

Instrumental Case

The authors' experience of running a large programme of patient educators involved in psychiatric education over the past thirteen years has shown consistently positive student feedback. However, it's not only students that benefit. Patients report a better understanding of their illness, with improved self-esteem and a sense of increased empowerment (Wykurz and Kelly, 2002; Towle et al., 2010). Moreover, patient educators report being pleased to have the opportunity to help students improve their understanding of psychosocial aspects of illness and their communication skills, and, overall, to be able to 'give something back' via medical education (Stacy and Spencer, 1999). They value learning new skills, the appreciation shown by students, and the support they receive from the teaching team.

However, implementation of service-user involvement programmes in higher education remains inconsistent (Basset, 1999). Progress has predominantly been concentrated within physical health specialties, and especially more long-term conditions and Primary Care. This growth hasn't been replicated in psychiatry, where challenges have led to slow and often limited approaches, which tend to focus on the delivery of personal narratives and Q&As with groups of students. Whilst valuable in providing opportunities to explore the human experiences of mental illness and healthcare provision, this fails to replicate the opportunity for students to benefit from direct patient feedback on their skills.

Some of the reticence to employ lived experience in the educational arena may arise from a range of ethical and educational concerns about the impact on patient educators' mental health, as well as about the long-term educational impact on student learning.

Ethical Concerns

Engaging patients with lived experience in psychiatric education raises several ethical concerns. Revealing one's intimate personal narrative to students clearly involves the patient educator breaching their own confidentiality. Obtaining valid and informed consent becomes absolutely vital to ensure that participation is voluntary and that patient trainers disclose only what they feel comfortable with (Jha, 2009a; Towle et al., 2010).

A more pressing concern perhaps is the risk of retraumatising or triggering patient educators. Patient educators are often required to maintain a fine balance between the rewards of training the new generation of doctors and the stress of training using one's own lived experience (Towle et al., 2010; Wykurtz and Kelly, 2002). Indeed, while this raises concerns about the potential for exploitation, this needs to be viewed in the context of long-standing stigma against people with mental illness that poses a barrier to gainful employment (Felton and Stickley, 2004). This underlines the importance of having appropriate processes in place to address these concerns when setting up patient educator programmes.

Educational Concerns

Patient narratives, while powerful, are too individualistic to provide a representative and diverse learning experience (Towle et al., 2010; Felton and Stickley, 2004). It is the authors' experience that without formal recruitment programmes, certain groups for example, Black, Asian, and Minority Ethnic patients, children/adolescents, or people with intellectual disability are less likely to be involved in teaching – a point emphasised also by Tew et al. (2004). An important caveat for patient involvement is that, like other faculty, their involvement in the programme should be to facilitate the delivery of desired learning outcomes for students. Addressing this at induction so that patient educators understand the curricular objectives helps address concerns about patient educators having an axe to grind with service providers (Livingston and Cooper, 2004). While short-term feedback of patient educator programmes may be positive, longer-term data about the impact of such programmes on student attitudes, behaviours, and clinical practice is largely lacking, particularly in psychiatry (Jha, 2009a).

The Derby 'Expert Patient' Project (Practical Considerations)

There are several practical considerations involved in setting up a sustainable educational programme with patient involvement. This section shares the experience of Derby Psychiatry Teaching Unit (PTU) of running its Expert Patient Programme (EPP) over the last thirteen years.

1) Underlying Values

There are two key values that drive the EPP: firstly, an educational focus on providing learning *experiences* to students given that experiential learning promotes deeper learning. Increasing face-to-face contact (albeit virtually when appropriate) between students and patients/carers facilitates this experiential learning. Secondly, an aspiration to co-production: that is, recognising that collaboration is an important first step in that process. This has meant moving away from a tokenistic involvement of patients in training to a more embedded process whereby patient involvement is woven into most if not all aspects of curriculum design and delivery. Apart from 45+ EPs who are now involved in a range of training activities, the faculty also boasts two lived-experience development workers, including one of the authors of this chapter (SR).

2) Develop Policies and Protocols

Having a nominated project lead is vital in translating values into action. EPs are in receipt of services and some of them do experience relapses that require enhanced care. Ensuring that EPs' clinical care is prioritised and that the educational team maintains its professional boundaries requires there to be adequate safeguarding arrangements and escalation protocols in place. These need to be negotiated with care teams and other stakeholders in advance. EPs themselves benefit from a comprehensive induction. Having a large 'bank' of EPs ensures adequate rotation of EPs' involvement and helps prevent burnout or stress.

3) Educational Outcomes

Engaging EPs early on in the educational aspects of the programme leads to a shift in focus from their personal experience of care (whether good or bad) to the idea of channelling their experience to help deliver the requisite learning outcomes. Training in how to provide objective feedback and in basic supervision skills, in our experience, helps empower EPs in discharging their educational role. Building in post-session debriefs for EPs as well as students provides an avenue to deal with both educational and non-educational issues that may have arisen during the interview.

4) Funding Considerations

Clearly, running a good-quality programme involving expert patients does incur financial expense. However, when compared with the costs of other experiential learning methods for example, surgical manikins, this is surprisingly affordable. Moreover, teaching in health settings attracts a reasonable income for the provider institution. In the case of Derby PTU, ring-fencing this income for medical student education has enabled us to recruit the necessary complement of medical and nurse educators, along with patient educators, to run the programme in a sustainable fashion.

5) Quality Assurance

The hallmark of a good programme is its ability to adapt to feedback and changing circumstances to ensure that the highest quality of teaching is delivered to students. Detailed feedback is obtained from students and from EPs, and action on this feedback has led to progressive evolution of the EP programme.

How to Involve EPs

Expert Patient Interviews

Medical students in their first ever placement in psychiatry often feel intimidated, particularly at the thought of obtaining a detailed history that requires delving into people's personal lives. At Derby PTU, each medical student is offered the opportunity of at least two sessions with an EP where, in a safe and supportive environment, they can attempt the task of taking a history and conducting a mental state examination, and can even carry out a safety/risk assessment. At the end of the session, the EP provides the student with comprehensive feedback on their interviewing skills and suggestions on how to improve. For struggling students, further remedial sessions with EPs are available if needed. Student feedback suggests they appreciate direct feedback on their communication skills and empathy, as well as the opportunity to practice asking difficult and sensitive questions in a safe environment. The availability of more than one session provides formative assessment that enables students to improve their interview and therapeutic relationship building skills over the course of the placement.

Interactive Seminars and Case-Based Learning

Weaving EP input into traditional forms of teaching such as lectures and seminars enriches them with a personal narrative. For instance, introducing a diagnosis-themed teaching session for depression with a real-person narrative provides a deeper, more humane understanding of the diagnosis. Co-presenting such a session with a clinician helps students draw links between presenting symptoms, the underlying pathophysiology, the rationale for various treatment strategies, the potential side effects, and the overall impact of symptoms as well as the treatment on the patient. This approach models person-centred care in providing a common platform for an EP to bring in their lived-experience expertise and for a clinician to bring in their professional clinical expertise to help students gain a broader and deeper understanding of the subject. EP input in other skills-focussed sessions, such as simulated OSCE-style task groups, keeps the learning grounded in real-life experience. Seminars on niche topics such as mental health law may also be developed with EP input.

Expert Patient Clinics

In a more recent development in the wake of the pandemic, EP clinics have been devised as an alternative to traditional outpatient clinics. Students attend a mock clinic (currently virtually/online), observe the clinical supervisor interview the EP, and subsequently have the opportunity to practise their interview skills under supervision. Feedback from both the EP and the clinical supervisor helps complete the learning loop for students.

Curricular Design, Development, and Assessment

There is a growing realisation that EPs have a valuable contribution to make to curricular design by ensuring that a person-centred focus is maintained in discussions about the standards that students/trainees need to attain at various points in their medical career.

Box 2.3.1 Take-Home Messages

1) Patient involvement in psychiatric (and medical) education has significant educational benefits for students, modelling person-centred care and building therapeutic relationship building skills.
2) Adequate planning and funding is needed to ensure that patient involvement in training is not tokenistic.
3) Advancing co-production principles in education should lead to the involvement of Expert Patients in all aspects of training and assessment.

Similarly, EPs' contribution in the assessment arena has largely been confined to formative assessments. Novel assessment strategies that allow for joint clinician/EP assessors may pave the way for the evaluation of students' capability of providing person-centred care.

References

Barrows, H. S. (1993). An overview of the uses of standardized patients for teaching and evaluating clinical skills. *AAMC, Academic Medicine*, **68** (6): 443–51.

Basset, T. (1999). Involving service users in training. *CARE*, 7: 5–11.

Byren, L., Happell, B., Welch, T., and Moxham, LJ. (2013). Things you can't learn from books: Teaching recovery from a lived experience perspective. *International Journal of Mental Health Nursing*, 22: 192–204.

Cleland, J. A., Abe, K., and Rethans, J.-J. (2009). The use of simulated patients in medical education: AMEE Guide No 42. *Medical Teacher*, **31** (6): 477–86.

Department of Health (1999). The National Service Framework for Mental Health. Available at: https://assets.publishing .service.gov.uk/government/uploads/system/ uploads/attachment_data/file/198051/ National_Service_Framework_for_Mental_ Health.pdf.

Department of Health (2001). *The Expert Patient: A New Approach to Chronic Disease Management for the 21st Century*. London: Department of Health.

Felton, A. and Stickley, T. (2004). Pedagogy, power and service user involvement. *Journal of Psychiatric and Mental Health Nursing*, **11**: 89–98.

Five Year Forward View for Mental Health (2016) – A report from the independent Mental Health Taskforce to the NHS in England. [online] NHSE. Available at: https:// www.england.nhs.uk/wp-content/uploads/ 2016/02/Mental-Health-Taskforce-FYFV-final.pdf (accessed 14 Nov. 2020).

Hojat, M., Vergare, M. J., Maxwell, K., et al. (2009). The devil is in the third year: A longitudinal study of erosion of empathy in medical school. *Academic medicine: Journal of the Association of American Medical Colleges* [online] **84** (9): 1182–91. Available at: www.ncbi.nlm.nih.gov/pubmed/19707055 (accessed 12 Dec. 2019).

Jha, V., Quinton, N. D., Bekker, H. L., Roberts, T. E. (2009a). Strategies and interventions for the involvement of real patients in medical education: A systematic review. *Medical Education*, **43**: 10–20.

Jha, V., Quinton, N. D., Bekker, H. L., Roberts, T. E. (2009b). What educators and students really think about using patients as teachers in medical education: A qualitative study. *Medical Education*, **43**: 449–56.

Lai, M. M. Y., Roberts, N., Mohebbi, M., and Martin, J. (2020). A randomised controlled trial of feedback to improve patient satisfaction and consultation skills in medical students. *BMC Medical Education*, **20** (1): 277.

Livingston, G. and Cooper, C. (2004). User and carer involvement in mental health training. *Advances in Psychiatric Treatment*, **10**: 85–92.

Mental Health and Social Exclusion. (2004). Available at: www.centreformental health.org.uk/sites/default/files/mental_ health_and_social_exclusion.pdf.

National Collaborating Centre for Mental Health (NCCMH). (2019). Working Well Together: Evidence and Tools to Enable Co-production in Mental Health Commissioning. London: National Collaborating Centre for Mental Health. Available at: www.rcpsych.ac.uk/docs/default-source/improving-care/nccmh/working-well-together/working-well-together—evidence-and-tools-to-enable-co-production-in-mental-health-commissioning.pdf?sfvrsn=4e2924c1_2 (accessed 26 March 2022).

Osler, W. (1901). Books and Men. *Boston Medical and Surgical Journal*, **144**: 60–1.

Royal College of Psychiatrists. (2018). Person-centred care: implications for training in psychiatry, RCPsych College Report CR215. Available at: www.rcpsych.ac.uk/docs/default-source/improving-care/better-mh-policy/college-reports/college-report-cr215.pdf? sfvrsn=7863b905_2 (accessed 24 May 2021).

Royal College of Psychiatrists. (2017). Core Values for Psychiatrists. RCPsych College

Report CR204. Available at: www
.rcpsych.ac.uk/docs/default-source/
improving-care/better-mh-policy/college-
reports/college-report-cr204.pdf?sfvrsn=
5e4ff507_2 (accessed 24 May 2021).

Stacy, R. and Spencer, J. (1999). Patients as
teachers: A qualitative study of patients'
views on their role in a community-based
undergraduate project. *Medical Education*,
33: 688–94.

Tew, J., Gell, C., and Foster, S. (2004). Learning
from experience: Involving service users and
carers in mental health education and
training. *Nottingham: Higher Education
Academy/NIMHE West Midlands/Trent
Workforce Development Confederation.*
Available at: www.swapbox.ac.uk/692/1/

learning-from-experience-whole-guide.pdf
(accessed 26 March 2022).

Towle, A. and Godolphin, W. (2009). Patients as
teachers: Promoting their authentic and
autonomous voices. *The Clinical Teacher*, **12**:
149–54.

Towle, A., Bainbridge, L., Godolphin, W., et al.
(2010). Active patient involvement in the
education of health professionals. *Medical
Education*, **44**, 64–74.

Towle, A., Brown, H., Hofely, C., et al. (2014).
The expert patient as teacher: An
interprofessional health mentors
programme. *The Clinical Teacher*, **11**: 301–6.

Wykurz, G. and Kelly, D. (2002). Developing the
role of patients as teachers: Literature review.
BMJ, **325**: 818–21.

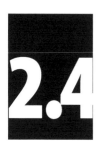

Assessment of Undergraduates in Psychiatry

Professor Brian Lunn

Introduction

Assessment in medical education is going through a period of change. Such episodes of change occur every few years, reflecting changes in underlying theory. Such 'tectonic' changes can be significant and, whilst initially slow, can lead to significant change in the end. If this was the only factor it would be significant, but there are two other factors at play in the United Kingdom. The first is the shift to the delivery of a national Medical Licensing Assessment (MLA) (Stephenson, 2017; The General Medical Council, 2020). This will inevitably have an impact not just on how students learn, but also on how they are taught. The other fact has been, and continues to be, the COVID pandemic. It would be naïve to view changes that have occurred to support education and assessment in this period as being a temporary aberration. They are likely to have a long-lasting impact even if, as is hoped, the impact of COVID is limited.

Conventionally, when reviewing assessment methodologies, writers tend to split the topic into knowledge, skill, and professionalism assessments. There are, however, two significant issues with this approach:

1. These are not discrete entities
2. These categories do not accurately relate to what the assessments, so labelled, actually deliver.

After considering the purpose of assessment, types of assessment will be covered under the headings 'Written Assessment' and 'Clinical Assessment', before moving on to the Medical Licensing Assessment (MLA) and post-COVID changes.

Purpose

Who is Assessment For?

Originally, assessment was primarily focussed on institutional requirements. Examinations were designed to assess whether a candidate had met the institution's standard and was considered a 'suitable' person to be awarded that institution's qualification. This continues to this day, particularly for non-professional undergraduate courses. It would be a mistake to think that this doesn't apply to medicine. In much of the early discussion around the MLA (covered later in this chapter) the need to maintain institutional standards was eminent. The central role of the institution continues into the postgraduate arena with qualifications such as the MRCPsych, albeit with regulatory oversight.

This brings us to the second important stakeholder, and an increasingly important one in medicine: the regulator. The General Medical Council (GMC) and other national regulators have long set out the standards for what is expected of undergraduate education. These cover both teaching and assessment. The regulator, in medicine, acts as a proxy for the profession, the government, and the public.

The final (and potentially the most important) group is learners. This epitomises an arguable dichotomy between assessment *of* learning versus assessment *for* learning. It is entirely feasible that these coexist in assessments. It should be essential that they do. In medicine this is important as students move from directed undergraduate learning to becoming increasingly independent learners in the postgraduate world.

Assessment Of or For Learning

Assessment of learning focusses on categorisation of learners. This can be on a continuum, a ranking assessment, or by determining whether a candidate is above or below a cut: a mastery assessment. In much of medicine, assessments are designed to make a mastery decision, often phrased around concepts of 'competence' or 'capability'. Assessments designed for this purpose are not good at distinguishing between levels of ability. To understand the difference between the two it can be helpful to use an analogy comparing the long jump and the high jump. In the long jump the athlete's performance is defined as the distance from the forward edge of the take-off board to the impression, closest to the take-off board, that they make in the landing pit. This reflects how ranking exams are graded. In the high jump what matters is clearing the bar. It doesn't matter how far above the bar the athlete is. This is analogous with a mastery level examination. These methodological differences make it difficult to rank students in mastery style examinations.

In psychiatry, as with all specialities, the relative proportion of psychiatric assessment items will impact on the degree to which an ability in our field contributes to ranking or mastery decisions.

In assessment for learning, whilst mastery or ranking decisions may be made, there is significant weight given to ensuring information from the assessment is delivered to candidates to allow them to drive their learning appropriately. Big, high-stakes, summative examinations typically do not do this. What is needed is an opportunity to diagnose and then repair. If a student receives timely information allowing them to identify their particular learning needs and address them, there is a shift to assessment for learning. Progress testing is one such approach (Wrigley et al., 2012). A progress test is usually administered to all students at the same time and at regular intervals (usually two to four times a year) throughout the entire course. Test content is drawn from the entire medical curriculum up to graduation, regardless of the students' point in the programme. The students' performance through this repeated testing allows charting of their progress towards the intended outcome of the course (graduation).

Assessing Psychiatry in Undergraduate Medical Education

Newble has shown that unforeseen and unintended consequences of assessment in a curriculum can be to drive student learning in undesirable ways (Newble, 2016). If psychiatry is not a core subject, with equal weight at assessment, students will value it less (Lunn, 2015, 2011). Psychiatry will only be given proportionate emphasis if we, as psychiatrists, seek engagement and leadership roles in assessment.

Unfortunately, psychiatry can be seen, particularly in clinical examinations, as 'difficult to assess'. If van der Vleuten's utility equation (Van Der Vleuten, 1996) is considered in its entirety this argument can be challenged, as educational impact is an essential component of assessment deign. Psychiatry, with its focus on complex patient interactions and the need to take an holistic view of the patient, represents a good model for assessment. As discussed later, post-COVID changes to assessment may give our speciality a leadership edge.

Written Assessments

Written assessments are typically represented as testing a 'knowledge' domain. As psychiatrists, however, we should be sceptical about any assessment mapping to a single domain. After all, we know that cognitive tests require a number of processes for each test, including, at the very least, language and comprehension skills. For this chapter, written assessments will be considered under two separate headings: 'Selected Item Assessments' and 'Constructed Item Assessments'.

Selected Item Assessments

In this form of assessment candidates select an answer from a provided list of options. Common forms of selected item assessments include:

- True/False questions
- Multiple-Choice Questions (MCQ)
- Extended Matching Items (EMI)
- Single Best Answer (SBA)

The format for each is broadly similar: a clinical stem followed by a question, and then an option list that will include the desired answer(s) and a number of distractors. The differing forms use these in different ways.

True/False questions have been largely abandoned in the United Kingdom for testing medical students. They are, however, used in other countries' medical schools (Cohen-Schotanus and van der Vleuten, 2010). This format rewards guessing and, potentially, risk taking. This is frequently controlled for by use of negative marking for incorrect answers or by adjusting the pass mark to control for guessing.

Well-constructed MCQs and SBAs have in common a clinical stem that contains the information a candidate needs to come to a conclusion on the theme tested and then the question on that theme. They are then presented with four or five options. In the MCQ there will be one correct answer. In the SBA there will be more than one 'correct' answer, but one will be the 'best' answer.

The problem inherent in this design is that it can be difficult to come up with a sufficient number of likely options to serve as realistic distractors. Typically, there may be one or more options that can be rapidly dismissed, leaving the candidate to choose from fewer options (Kilgour and Tayyaba, 2016).

Constructing good items is a difficult process and can result in items with a limited shelf life. This refers to the possibility that in the time between creation and examination there is a change in potential answers. Examples of this would be emerging treatment guidelines or changes in diagnostic criteria. This can, perversely, reward the poorer candidate who may be less aware of up-to-date guidance, diagnostic criteria, or theoretical models.

Table 2.4.1 The four elements of a well-constructed extended matching item (EMI) assessment

Element	Content
The theme	This is the topic that will be assessed by the stems and is the unifying element of the options list. Examples might be psychopathological terms, laboratory investigations or results, drugs from a class, diagnostic terms, etc.
The option list	This provides the various possible answers for the stems. While the number of options can vary, it is important that there is uniformity of theme, and that there are sufficient options to allow valid testing of knowledge. Questions can be made 'more difficult' by increasing the number of options (providing that there is uniformity of option type) or decreasing the degree of difference between options. Options can be single words, phrases, or numerical values such as 'results'. It is important that there is a common structure as well as a common theme.
The lead statement	A single lead statement should be used for all stems in each individual EMI to provide direction and identify the relationship between the stems and the option list. The lead statement can require the candidate to select more than one option or to order the options in some way. It is vital to give explicit directions as EMIs with non-specific lead statements can create ambiguity.
The stems	In psychiatry, perhaps the most useful form of theme is a clinical vignette, which describes a patient in a clinical situation. If carefully constructed, these can be used to draw relationships between basic and clinical sciences and test knowledge of subjects such as descriptive psychopathology or application of diagnoses. In common with other components of EMIs, stems in each EMI should be similar in structure to minimise guessing.

Other examples of poor questions include where item authors only use a stem to present a simple 'select one from' question or to present questions relating to an eponymous theory. The latter is an issue particularly when social sciences or psychological issues are being assessed.

Well-constructed EMIs follow the model set out in Table 2.4.1.

As can be seen, the issue can be in deriving enough realistic distractors of the same type. All too often a variety of different types of distractors (e.g. drugs and investigations) are used. Again, this reduces the likelihood of a number of distractors being selected and improves the chances of guessing an answer correctly.

At heart, however, for those practised in cognitive testing it can be recognised that having a good recognition memory is at the core of performing well in selected items.

Constructed Item Assessments

The difference between recognition and recall memory is at the heart of the differences between selected and constructed items. In the latter the candidate is required to write the correct answer. Formats include:

- Essays
- Short Answer Questions (SAQ)
- Very Short Answer items (VSA)

As with selected items, these assessments can map to more than simple knowledge of a topic. Essays also assess literacy, the ability to construct an argument or present cogent data, and (possibly) legibility of handwriting (along with grammar, syntax, and spelling). In timed environments this can result in indirect discrimination affecting those for whom the exam is not set in their first language or those with specific learning differences such as dyslexia, dyspraxia, or dysgraphia. What is being assessed is, therefore, not just candidates' knowledge of the topic, but also their skill in writing essays. This may be appropriate, but at undergraduate level and in timed assessments it is of limited value.

Essays can be as reliable as other forms of assessment (Stalenhoef-Halling et al., 1990), but marking them is time intensive, and it is unlikely that institutions would reach an acceptable reliability standard taking into account logistical matters. This reduction in reliability significantly impacts the validity of essays in the undergraduate setting.

SAQs have greater utility, being more amenable to marking, including team marking, which enhances reliability. They do, however, carry the issues that affect essays vis-à-vis indirect discrimination. In common with other assessment formats, there may be the issue of whether candidates correctly infer what the question-setter was looking for. Dealing with what may well be a reasonable interpretation of a question that doesn't match a model answer is difficult in post hoc exam analysis.

A newer form of assessment item is the VSA. Like the other constructed answer items, it benefits from manual input marking, but this is linked to computational methods that significantly decrease the marking load and decrease inter-rater variability.

Like SBAs, VSAs consist of a clinical stem followed by a question. Where this differs is that candidates do not select an answer but have to write one in. Questions are constructed so that the answer required is one to five words in length (hence, 'very short') (Sam et al., 2019). The exam is delivered electronically, and in setting the question the author identifies the likely correct and incorrect responses. Computerised marking will automatically flag all of these and mark accordingly. Responses that do not reflect the model responses are then reviewed manually. If a 'correct' answer that was not included in the original model is identified, then all candidates providing this response are automatically marked accordingly and the response saved for future use of this item. A similar approach is applied to unexpected incorrect responses.

Possible benefits of this format include being responsive to changes in guidance and understanding, being relatively light on marker effort, and driving different learning styles (Sam et al., 2016). Sam et al. (2019), looking at medical students across the United Kingdom in a pilot of VSAs, compared how the test cohort answered a series of VSAs and best-of-five SBAs with identical stems and questions. Comparing the facility of responses in SBA and VSA format showed a significantly higher facility in candidates' responses to the SBA format, indicating a significant cue rate. The psychometric evidence for this form of assessment is robust (Sam et al., 2018) and has the potential to be a better form of assessment for assessing psychiatry, where finding sufficient robust distractors can be an issue.

In assessing knowledge of psychiatry, there are a number of factors that need to be considered. Emerging utility evidence would suggest that there would be benefit from shifting to the current prevalent selected item model to use of VSA constructed items.

Clinical Assessments

Assessment of clinical skills is key to undergraduate medical student programmes. The trend over recent years is to move to increasingly standardised examinations. This is understandable with pressures to defend decisions and reassure the regulator, but it carries with it issues.

The Objective Structured Clinical Examination (OSCE) has become the standardised format, to such an extent that some recent papers have assumed that schools only use this as a clinical examination format (Devine et al., 2015). The picture is much more complex, with medical schools using a combination of Workplace Based Assessment (WPBA) formats and alternative, longer format assessments such as the Modified Observed Structured Long Examination Record (MOSLER) (Wright et al., 2009). This allows structured but less standardised assessments where there is greater validity.

The historical dominant use of high stakes summative examination models leads to in vitro assessment models being the dominant format in UK medical schools. Use of in vivo formats is more commonly seen in the postgraduate arena, particularly beyond core training, but there is a strong argument to increase their use in the undergraduate arena.

In Vitro Assessments

In vitro assessments have long had a prominent role in undergraduate assessment. Originally this was in the long- and short-case formats or scenario-based vivas. This shifted, beginning in the 1970s (Harden et al., 1975; Tyrer, 2005) to increasing use of the OSCE. It wasn't until some time after the development of the first OSCE that it was used as a tool in psychiatry, although its use has developed over subsequent years (Hodges et al., 2014). One of the challenges in using OSCE stations in a psychiatric setting is that of developing a marking system that reflects good practice. Hodges et al. (1999) have shown that a checklist-based approach can reward less experienced candidates, whilst a more global approach rewards the more experienced candidate. In general, for undergraduate OSCEs, wherein a range of clinical disciplines are assessed, it can be difficult to ensure that marking schemes that reflect good psychiatric clinical practice are used. The alternative can lead to poorer skill development.

The use of other, longer formats can add validity without loss of reliability (Wass et al., 2001; Wass and Van Der Vleuten, 2004) and, with the ability to bring together an integrated approach, moves the assessment higher up Miller's Pyramid as well as fitting a psychiatric case more accurately (Miller, 1990).

In constructing clinical scenarios, a particular approach is required. Whilst tempting to anonymise a real patient's story, this will lead to the assessment objective being secondary to the role written. It is vital that the process is the opposite of this. The objective of the assessment comes first, and then the role is constructed to facilitate this (Bateman et al., 2013).

One important matter to consider in constructing scenarios for clinical assessments is that authors often conform to what is familiar – that is, they are more likely to write scenarios based on their personal experience. This leads to biases, such as a likelihood that role-players' ethnicities match the author's, or that the role tends towards higher socio-economic groups. Using patient representatives to support role development can broaden the roles written and increase authenticity. The RCPsych has made use of patients in assessment design and this is also well advanced in health research; there are good resources available from the likes of the National Institute for Health Research ('NIHR | INVOLVE').

In Vivo Assessments

Feedback and evaluation of performance in real clinical environments, outside the artificial reality of in vitro assessments, is increasingly recognised as important in the development of medical students (Ramani et al., 2018). WPBAs are an important postgraduate tool and aim to assess the 'top' hierarchical component of 'Does', as identified by Miller (1990). This, along with the identification that using global marking more accurately identifies expertise, is increasing focus on the validity of subjective judgements and assessment in clinical environments (Hodges, 2013). Indeed, there is a global shift in the academic field towards assessment of competence (Van Der Vleuten, 1996) and the need to develop integrated assessments that recognise the value of formative elements in assessment (Konopasek et al., 2016) and competency-based portfolios (Oudkerk Pool et al., 2018).

Whilst relevant for all medical specialities, a particular benefit in psychiatry is students seeing 'real' patients. These patients do not adhere to a script, act in a predictable manner, or respond to predetermined cues. Taking histories and examining the multitude of individual presentations is a critical skill for all clinicians and so using in vivo assessments in clinical environments adds real value to assessment.

As we gradually shift towards what Hodges (2013) has called a post-psychometric era, and, as in vivo assessment tools are developed (see section: 'Post-COVID assessment'), we in psychiatry have an opportunity to take a lead. The use of computation-psychometric analysis (von Davier et al., 2019) of large, unstructured data sets will likely lead to a shift away from the big final exam to more granular 'real-life' assessments – something that will better reflect our clinical practice.

The Medical Licensing Assessment

Internationally, there has been increasing focus on national licensing assessment. National licensing assessments are already in place in Canada, the USA, Switzerland, most ASEAN countries, China, and, imminently, the United Kingdom (Swanson and Roberts, 2016). There are several drivers here, which include perceived differences between UK medical schools (McCrorie and Boursicot, 2009) and the desire to control safe access to the workforce for international graduates (Stephenson and Dickson, 2016). For UK medical students, those graduating in the cohort for the academic year 2024–25 will be required by the GMC to sit and pass an MLA. This will constitute part of their medical degree and will be a requirement for them to join the medical register.

Aside from the drive to be seen to regulate, there has been a view that there are differing standards across UK medical schools, although the research looking at data from common content in written finals examined the views of standard-setting groups, across medical schools, on a limited number of items, rather than whole exams items (Taylor et al., 2017).

Not all medical schools have a clearly labelled psychiatric element at Finals. Regardless of the intent, it is inevitable that having the MLA as a graduating requirement will lead to students focussing on it – a foreseeable but unintended consequence. If psychiatry is not a core requirement in all medical schools' final exams, then it will inevitably be given lower priority by revising students.

Post-COVID Assessment

Whilst, at the time of writing, we remain with restrictions on daily life and restrictions on teaching in university settings, it is unlikely that, following the pandemic, teaching and assessment will remain the same. With the need for distanced assessment there has been renewed attention paid to novel assessment modalities. This has included taking a more programmatic approach, looking at the whole range of assessment types to focus in-person assessment where it was needed most (as carried out in Newcastle University Medical School) to novel teleconference assessments. One concern is that these latter assessments can take the format of a case-based discussion, asking what students would do – very much a lower-order assessment (according to Miller's pyramid) compared to in vivo or standard in vitro clinical assessments. Psychiatry is better placed than many disciplines to look at this in a fresh light. Clinical practice has had to shift to telemedicine in many cases. Constructing clinical assessment around such scenarios therefore reflects clinical reality and has the possibility of constructing in vivo assessments. It should not be forgotten, however, that these are resource intensive and have the potential to increase indirect socio-economic discrimination due to students' varied access to high-quality IT equipment and/or fast reliable broadband.

Summary

The academic field of assessment research and development is developing rapidly. Drivers include environmental factors (regulation such as the MLA, the pandemic, etc.) and technical factors (research evidence and the development of computational psychometrics). What has not changed is the need to ensure that psychiatry is considered as an essential component of final assessments, and that in curricula development the assessment of our speciality is built in from the outset.

References

Bateman, J., Allen, M., Samani, D., Kidd, J., and Davies, D. (2013). Virtual patient design: Exploring what works and why. A grounded theory study. *Medical Education.* **47**, 595–606.

Cohen-Schotanus, J. and van der Vleuten, C. P. M. (2010). A standard setting method with the best performing students as point of reference: Practical and affordable. *Medical Teacher.* **32**, 154–60.

von Davier, A. A., Deonovic, B., Yudelson, M., Polyak, S. T., and Woo, A. (2019). Computational psychometrics approach to holistic learning and assessment systems. *Frontiers in Education.* **4**, 1–12.

Devine, O. P., Harborne, A. C., and McManus, I. C. (2015). Assessment at UK medical schools varies substantially in volume, type and intensity and correlates with postgraduate attainment. *BMC Medical Education.* **15**, 1–13.

General Medical Council (2020). Medical Licensing Assessment [Online] Available at: www.gmc-uk.org/education/medical-licensing-assessment (accessed 19 January 2021).

Harden, R. M. G., Downie, W. W., Stevenson, M., and Wilson, G. M. (1975). Assessment of clinical competence using objective structured examination. *British Medical Journal.* **1**, 447–51.

Hodges, B. (2013). Assessment in the post-psychometric era: learning to love the subjective and collective. *Medical Teacher.* **35**, 564–8.

Hodges, B. D., Hollenberg, E., McNaughton, N., Hanson, M. D., and Regehr, G. (2014). The psychiatry OSCE: A 20-year retrospective. *Academic Psychiatry.* **38**, 26–34.

Hodges, B., Regehr, G., McNaughton, N., Tiberius, R., and Hanson, M. (1999). OSCE checklists do not capture increasing levels of expertise. *Academic Medicine.* **74**, 1129–34.

Kilgour, J. M. and Tayyaba, S. (2016). An investigation into the optimal number of distractors in single-best answer exams. *Advances in Health Sciences Education.* **21**, 571–85.

Konopasek, L., Norcini, J., and Krupat, E. (2016). Focusing on the formative: Building an assessment system aimed at student growth and development. *Academic Medicine.* **91** (11): 1492–7.

Lunn, B. (2011). Recruitment into psychiatry: An international challenge. *Australian and New Zealand Journal of Psychiatry.* **45**, 805–7.

Lunn, B. (2015). 'Education in Psychiatry', in: Bhugra, D. (Ed.), *International Encyclopedia of the Social & Behavioral Sciences.* Elsevier, pp. 185–93.

McCrorie, P. and Boursicot, K. A. M. (2009). Variations in medical school graduating examinations in the United Kingdom: Are clinical competence standards comparable? *Medical Teacher.* **31**: 223–9.

Miller, G. E. (1990). The assessment of clinical skills/competence/performance. *Academic Medicine.* **65**: S63–S67.

Newble, D. (2016). Revisiting 'The effect of assessments and examinations on the learning of medical students'. *Medical Education.* **50**: 498–501.

NIHR | INVOLVE [Online] Available at: www .nihr.ac.uk/health-and-care-professionals/ engagement-and-participation-in-research/ involve-patients.htm (accessed 19 January 2021).

Oudkerk Pool, A., Govaerts, M. J. B., Jaarsma, D. A. D. C., and Driessen, E. W. (2018). From aggregation to interpretation: How assessors judge complex data in a competency-based portfolio. *Advances in Health Sciences Education.* **23**, 275–87.

Ramani, S., Könings, K. D., Ginsburg, S., van der Vleuten, and C. P. M. (2018). Twelve tips to promote a feedback culture with a growth mind-set: Swinging the feedback pendulum from recipes to relationships. *Medical Teacher.* **10**, 1–7.

Sam, A. H., Field, S. M., Collares, C. F., et al. (2018). Very-short-answer questions: Reliability, discrimination and acceptability. *Medical Education.* **52**, 447–55.

Sam, A. H., Hameed, S., Harris, J., and Meeran, K. (2016). Validity of very short answer versus single best answer questions for undergraduate assessment. *BMC Medical Education.* **16**, 10–13.

Sam, A. H., Westacott, R., Gurnell, M., Wilson, R., Meeran, K., and Brown, C. (2019). Comparing single-best-answer and very-short-answer questions for the assessment of applied medical knowledge in 20 UK medical schools: Cross-sectional study. *British Medical Journal Open.* **9**, 1–7.

Stalenhoef-Halling, B., van der Vleuten, C., Jaspers, T., and Fiolet, J. (1990). 'The feasibility, acceptability and reliability of openended questions in a problem based learning curriculum', in Hiemstra, R., Scherpbier, A., and Zwiestra, R. (Eds.), *Teaching and Assessing Clinical Competence.* Groningen: Boekwerk, pp. 1020–31.

Stephenson, T. (2017). Medical licensing assessment will keep us ahead of the field. *British Medical Journal.* **356**: j594.

Stephenson, T. and Dickson, N. (2015). Working together to develop a medical licensing assessment: Findings from our engagement with UK medical schools. [Online] Available at: www .gmc-uk.org/-/media/documents/Report_ of_MLA_visits_to_medical_schools_v1 .0.pdf_68172878.pdf (accessed 24 March 2022).

Swanson, D. B. and Roberts, T. E. (2016). Trends in national licensing examinations in medicine. *Medical Education.* **50**, 101–14.

Taylor, C. A., Gurnell, M., Melville, C. R., Kluth, D. C., Johnson, N., and Wass, V. (2017). Variation in passing standards for graduation-level knowledge items at UK medical schools. *Medical Education.* **51**, 612–20.

Tyrer, S. (2005). 'Development of the OSCE: A College perspective', in Rao, R. (Ed.), *OSCEs in Psychiatry.* London: Royal College of Psychiatrists/Gaskill, pp. 14–23.

Van Der Vleuten, C. P. M. (1996). The
assessment of professional competence:
Developments, research and practical
implications. *Advances in Health Sciences
Education.* **1**, 41–67.

Wass, V., Jones, R., and Van Der Vleuten, C.
(2001). Standardized or real patients to test
clinical competence? The long case revisited.
Medical Education. **35**, 321–5.

Wass, V. and Van Der Vleuten, C. (2004). The
long case. *Medical Education.* **38**, 1176–80.

Wright, S., Bradley, P., Jones, S., and Barton, R.
(2009). 'Generalisability study of a new Finals
examination component – The MOSLER', in
AMEE 2009. Málaga: Association for Medical
Education in Europe, p. S106.

Wrigley, W., Van Der Vleuten, C. P.,
Freeman, A., and Muijtjens, A. (2012).
A systemic framework for the progress
test: Strengths, constraints and issues:
AMEE Guide No. 71. *Medical Teacher.* **34**,
683–97.

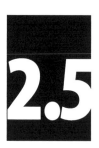

2.5 Beyond the Undergraduate Core Curriculum

Dr Julie Langan Martin and Dr Daniel Martin

High-quality psychiatric teaching of medical students is essential to enable high-quality care as well as for recruitment to speciality. This chapter explores some of the additional structured opportunities, which may be useful for educational supervisors to discuss with medical students interested in a career in psychiatry.

The Royal College of Psychiatrists

The Royal College of Psychiatrists (RCPsych) plays an important role in undergraduate medical education and offers numerous resources and opportunities which may be helpful to interested medical students and educational supervisors.

One example, for those interested in medical education, is the undergraduate education forum, which has a role in strategic planning between medical schools and the College. The group has a role in contributing to national policy on undergraduate medical education. Each medical school has one representative at the forum (usually the lead for psychiatry, or their deputy). In certain instances, the forum may create subgroups, which may require additional members. More information is available here: www.rcpsych.ac.uk/become-a-psychiatrist/supporting-medical-students?searchTerms=education%20forum.

The College has also developed the PDF download 'Choose Psychiatry Guidance for Medical Schools' (Choose Psychiatry, 2019), which highlighted four key recommendations for improving students' experience of psychiatry:

1. Excellence in teaching
2. Quality placements
3. Leadership
4. Enriching experiences, which may include electives, specialist study modules, psychiatric societies, and summer schools.

There are further opportunities for interested psychiatrists to get involved with the Choose Psychiatry activities offered by the College. For example, the Choose Psychiatry in Scotland (CPS) Committee (formerly the Scottish Training and Recruitment Group STaRG) has several projects and roles for psychiatrists interested in recruitment.

For interested medical students, there are several resources available online that describe a day in the life of a psychiatrist. These resources highlight the variety and multidisciplinary nature of the work undertaken within psychiatry and are a helpful resource for students interested in a career in psychiatry. Recent posts include 'What it's like being redeployed from psychiatry to A&E during a pandemic', 'We must work together', and 'What makes a great psychiatrist? Four core skills every trainee psychiatrist needs.' You can read these on the RCPsych Website: www.rcpsych.ac.uk/news-and-features/blogs.

Within the College, medical students can sign up (without cost) to become an associate of the RCPsych. This gives them electronic access to the *BJPsych*, *BJPsych Bulletin*, and *BJPsych Advances* journals, as well as copies of the biannual *Associate* magazine. Medical student associates may also apply for bursaries to attend certain RCPsych conferences and in some instances free places are available to medical students.

Psychiatry Societies

Most medical schools will have a Psychiatric Society or PsychSoc. There is a list of PsychSocs available for UK medical schools on the RCPscyh website. Most have a Facebook page or Twitter profile. There are good opportunities for enthusiastic psychiatrists to speak at events organised by the local psychiatric society, which may be a helpful starting point for medical students interested in psychiatry.

Summer and/or Autumn Schools

Another way to encourage students interested in psychiatry is through the running of Summer and/or Autumn schools. These events tend to be organised jointly by locality medical school(s), PsychSoc(s), and the RCPsych. These helpful programmes typically run on an annual basis and often provide a good overview of the diversity of the careers available in psychiatry. It may be possible for these to be run remotely as webinars in response to the COVID-19 pandemic.

Electives

Medical schools usually offer one or two elective placements to their students. This is often in the final or penultimate year of study. Typically, these are blocks of study which last between four and eight weeks and allow more in-depth experience of a particular area. Psychiatric electives are a good opportunity to engage students in psychiatry. Opportunities to study abroad can provide additional insights into cross-cultural psychiatric illness and practice. A wide range of sub-specialities within psychiatry provide excellent opportunities for student learning during an elective placement. Examples include perinatal psychiatry, child and adolescent psychiatry, forensic psychiatry, and older adult psychiatry, amongst others. The apprenticeship model used within clinical placements often works well for students on electives, and exposure to multidisciplinary team (MDT) working is equally important. Exposure to MDT working allows students to feel like part of the team and allows good breadth and depth of learning experiences, as well as opportunities for triangulation in assessment.

Depending on the student's medical school and where you work, the practicalities of organising an elective will vary. For example, some universities encourage students to organise their own elective placement, write their own intended learning outcomes (ILOs), and decide on the form of assessment. Other universities provide an online list of electives that students can apply for using the relevant application form. In some cases, a fee is applied although, as noted, opportunities for financial support often exist through both the RCPsych and the Universities themselves. Many students are asked to write an elective report which they submit to their university as part of their assessment for their elective placements.

There are also third-party organisations which contain lists of available medical student electives. Although most universities and Royal Colleges do not endorse these websites, they can provide students with a helpful starting point when organising their elective. In some cases, student bursaries and prizes are available to help meet the cost of student's electives, at least in part.

If you wish to become involved in being an elective supervisor, it is worth contacting the Director of Electives (or equivalent) at your local university. From there, you will be able to discuss the best way to organise your elective placements.

Specialist Study Modules/Components

Specialist Study Modules (SSMs) or Specialist Study Components (SSCs) allow students to spend a fixed period (usually four to six weeks) exploring an area of interest that may also influence and inform future career choice. The second edition of Tomorrow's Doctors recognised that SSCs must allow students to 'consider potential career paths' (GMC, 2003, p. 18) and so SSCs and SSMs may act as an opportunity to recruit medical students to psychiatry.

Therefore, all medical schools offer SSMs and SSCs in psychiatry. Such SSMs or SSCs can be self-proposed by the student, pre-designed by the medical school, or pre-designed by the professional who leads the module. Data from the RCPsych Survey suggests that these modules can provide positive experiences for medical students and encourage recruitment to speciality.

Whilst there are many advantages in terms of specific interests and experiences offered by self-selected SSCs or SSMs, pre-existing or teacher-led modules are often more structured and directed. In increasingly busy and demanding clinical environments, medical students can be encouraged to join existing clinical teams to gain relevant experience. In some cases, students can become involved in quality improvement (QI) and audit projects. This can be helpful when considering one's own appraisal. Approaching your local medical school's student-selected-components/modules lead is a good place to start when considering proposing such a placement.

A diverse range of SSMs and SSCs can be undertaken by students, and several innovative modules can and have been developed. Some innovative SSC examples include: 'Madness and the Movies' (Datta, 2009) and 'Dark side of the Moon' (Adams, 2008).

Volunteering and Voluntary Organisations

Gordon Johnston

In addition to structured study options, students may also wish to consider seeking voluntary positions. This can enable them to gain more practical experience or greater direct interaction with people who have lived experience.

Many national and local voluntary organisations are structured as user-led charities, with boards comprised wholly or partially of their members. They carry out a wide range of roles, including advocacy and campaigning, providing direct services such as peer support initiatives, and they offer a range of opportunities for people with lived experience to support each other.

Voluntary organisations are usually reliant on grants and fundraising activities and will often offer volunteering positions, thereby providing opportunities to gain experience. These might include facilitating a support group, assisting in the development of new project ideas and funding bids, or providing direct support to people with lived experience in their activities.

Volunteering can be rewarding for the student, in terms of giving something directly to a charitable cause, and also extremely useful in developing skills and putting knowledge gained during study to practical use.

Intercalated Degrees

A number of intercalated degrees are available to medical students with an interest in psychiatry. Such degrees may include psychological medicine, psychology and behavioural science, neuroscience, and pharmacology. Less traditional, arts-based degrees such as medical literature, medical history, and journalism are also available. In some cases, linguistic degrees may even be possible. These requests are considered by several universities. For certain intercalated degrees medical students join the Honours year of a separate degree programme, whilst other programmes consist only of intercalating medical students. Some universities may provide a two-year intercalated degree programme resulting in a master's level degree.

Intercalated degrees provide an opportunity to look at a topic in depth and develop skills and understanding of research methods, and may give an advantage later in an individual's career. This being said, the departure from a medical school year can in some cases be unsettling and distracting. Historically, intercalated degrees have been open to students with academic and research-based interests, although their availability has broadened in recent years. Indeed, in many UK universities, an intercalated degree is now embedded within the medical curricula.

When choosing an intercalated degree, it is important for students to be clear and honest about their reasons and motivation for completing the degree. Many students may struggle with the diverse ways of working and the heavy burden of independent learning, as compared to a more directly taught medical curriculum. Intercalated degrees are for many students their first experience of literature searching, critical analysis, and less directed learning. It may be prudent to read some relevant background material prior to selecting and enrolling in an intercalated degree programme. Furthermore, there are several practical skills involved in intercalated degree programmes which are likely to be new but nonetheless interesting to prospective students. One example is laboratory work, which can be rewarding and challenging in equal measures. Similarly, neuroimaging can on the face of it seem relatively accessible, but the realities can be tricky. One other factor to consider is the gaining of new skills in ethics, which prospective students may wish to familiarise themselves with ahead of applying.

Postgraduate Study

There are many opportunities for further study available to postgraduate psychiatrists, both trainees and consultants. Most master's level degree programmes will consider applications from people who have obtained a medical degree. Therefore, the possibilities for postgraduate study are wide and varied.

For example, for those interested in medical education, there are opportunities to undertake a postgraduate certificate (PgCert), a postgraduate diploma (PgDip), or a master's level degree in learning and teaching (MEd). Others may be interested in developing legal skills, and there are opportunities where some may undertake a law degree (LLB).

For those interested in developing research skills, a Master of Public Health, a Master of Science (MSc), Master of Research (MRes) or indeed a Master of Philosophy (MPhil), may be undertaken. Many of these programmes of study can be taken part time, and increasingly many taught masters courses can be delivered online. Finally, for individuals who are considering an academic career, a higher degree such as a Doctor of Medicine (MD) or a Doctor of Philosophy (PhD) may be undertaken.

References

Adams, B. (2008). Dark side of the moon: A course in mental health and the arts. *Psychiatric Bulletin*. **32**: 227–9. https://doi.org/10.1192/pb.bp.107.016824.

Choose Psychiatry, Sept 2019. Available at: www.rcpsych.ac.uk/docs/default-source/become-a-psychiatrist/guidance-for-medical-schools-pdf.pdf?sfvrsn=20f46cae_14.

Datta, V. Madness and the movies: An undergraduate module for medical students. *Int Rev Psychiatry*. 2009 Jun; **21** (3): 261–6.

https://doi.org/10.1080/09540260902748001. PMID: 19459103.

GMC. (2003). *Tomorrow's Doctors: Outcomes and standards for undergraduate medical education.* General Medical Council. Available at: www.educacionmedica.net/pdf/documentos/modelos/tomorrowdoc.pdf (accessed 24 March 2022).

PsySoc List: www.rcpsych.ac.uk/become-a-psychiatrist/med-students/psychsocs.

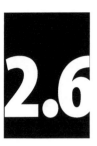

2.6

Supporting the Psychiatrists of Tomorrow

Zoé Mulliez

The psychiatrists of tomorrow need a unique skill set to provide the holistic care that people with mental illness need, including curiosity, a collaborative spirit, creativity, and the willingness to be intellectually challenged. A variety of initiatives exist to support all medical students in gaining the necessary interpersonal skills while further developing their scientific knowledge and medical expertise.

Those who have chosen psychiatry as a specialty know the breadth of career opportunities it offers. Any future doctor benefits from exposure to psychiatry, even if they decide to choose another career path. It is essential that the next generation of doctors is fully aware of both the importance of mental health for everyone and the positive difference that psychiatry makes to people's lives.

This chapter provides a non-exhaustive list of some of the initiatives currently available. Some are run by universities with support from the Royal College of Psychiatrists (RCPsych) and could be replicated across the country. We encourage all medical schools' leaders and undergraduate teaching leads in psychiatry to familiarise themselves with these innovative strategies and activities. These can be harnessed to raise awareness of psychiatry as a speciality and positively impact on future recruitment.

University Support

Psychiatry Societies ('PsychSocs')

First set up in 2005 by King's College London, psychiatry societies (also known as 'PsychSocs') are university societies promoting careers in psychiatry and raising the profile of mental health amongst all students. There are thirty-four PsychSocs at or affiliated to medical schools across the United Kingdom.

The RCPsych supports PsychSocs in different ways, such as organising the annual National Student Psychiatry Conference (hosted by a lead PsychSoc in partnership with the College, with around 100–200 delegates annually) and the national meeting of PsychSoc presidents. The College offers each PsychSoc £500 per year and has awarded a total of £83,437 in PsychSoc bursaries since 2013. Practical guidance on how to set up PsychSocs and how to run PsychSoc events can be found on the RCPsych website (see www.rcpsych.ac.uk/become-a-psychiatrist/med-students/psychsocs/setting-up-your-psychsoc and www.rcpsych.ac.uk/become-a-psychiatrist/med-students/psychsocs/how-to-run-psychsoc-events).

In developing the Choose Psychiatry guidance for medical schools (Mulliez, 2019), medical students suggested innovative ways to reach a wider audience and attract students who may not be interested in psychiatry in the first instance. One suggestion was to organise events exploring the interface between mental health and wider societal issues, such as human rights, sport, housing, employment, the arts, and even spirituality. When exposed to the importance of mental health to the wider society, the psychiatrists of tomorrow may be more likely to advocate for the need to move mental health into the mainstream of policy and practice.

Mentoring and Shadowing Programmes

Mentoring, shadowing, and coaching play crucial roles in developing and supporting the psychiatrists of tomorrow. Examples include 'PsychStart', a career-based mentoring scheme in Nottingham that allows medical students to experience what life as a psychiatrist is like, and the Psychiatry Early Experience Programme (PEEP), which offers students the opportunity to shadow core psychiatry trainees over their five years of training across a wide variety of specialties.

Extra-Curricular Courses

Many medical students have mentioned their lack of confidence to engage with people suffering from mental illness. While some students participate in various induction activities before they start their placement in psychiatry, others receive little to no preparation.

To address this, a group of psychiatrists run 'Extreme Psychiatry', an innovative course for Year 3 King's College London medical students. Designed to give all students the skills and confidence they need to help people with mental illness, the course also aims to decrease stigma.

Inspired by this scheme, three psychiatrists created 'Psychiatry Pitstop', a similar course that runs for six weeks twice a year and is accessible for free at the University of Leeds Medical School and Hull York Medical School. Tested over the last few years, the programme could easily be adapted and delivered in other universities.

Career enrichment courses (often referred to as 'summer', 'autumn', or 'winter' schools) bring together students who are considering a career in psychiatry for an intensive programme of lectures, debates, and networking opportunities. Students highlighted the benefits of meeting inspiring psychiatrists and leading researchers, as well as medical students from other medical schools with a similar interest in psychiatry.

Support Provided by the Royal College of Psychiatrists (RCPsych)

The Choose Psychiatry Campaign and Programme of Activities

The Choose Psychiatry media campaign is the first external digital marketing campaign the College has run, and it aims to promote psychiatry as a diverse, meaningful career that dramatically improves the lives of those living with serious mental illness. It includes a range of inspiring films available on a dedicated YouTube channel, which is followed by 7.63 k people.

As part of the campaign, the College produces a range of blogs and podcasts to inspire future doctors. It proactively engages with medical students in innovative ways online and via social media; at the time of writing, there are 4,820 people 'following' the Choose Psychiatry Twitter account. It also runs a hard-hitting news story every year to remind the public that we need to invest in psychiatry to ensure we can help more people access the right services at the right time.

The College also runs a wide Choose Psychiatry programme of activities to support school students, foundation doctors, trainees, and others to consider a career in psychiatry. Amongst its activities, it has set up Choose Psychiatry networks, with fifty-five active members supporting recruitment into psychiatry across the United Kingdom.

The latest figures demonstrate the positive impact the whole campaign (both the media campaign and the programme of activities) has had on recruitment, with nearly a 100% CT1 fill rate in England in 2019, compared to 67.3% in 2017 (Health Education England, 2020).

Student Associates and the Psych STAR Scheme

All medical students interested in a career in psychiatry can become 'Student Associates'. Associates can attend free events and get discounted rates to meet renowned international psychiatrists at the College's annual International Congress. They have free access to online training (through a resource called 'Trainees Online' or TrOn), free electronic access to a range of magazines, and discounted rates on all other RCPsych Publications. They also receive e-newsletters and copies of the biannual Associate magazine, *Future Psych*. As of July 2020, 3,793 medical students were Student Associates.

Designed by Professor Helen Bruce, Dr Declan Hyland, and Clare Wynn-Mackenzie, the 'Psych STAR' scheme goes further in providing support to medical students. For one year, successful applicants receive additional benefits, including mentoring, an induction evening at the College, free access to the International Congress, CPD and travel funds to be spent on courses, conferences, and learning materials, and free print copies of the RCPsych journals. Since its creation in 2019, twenty-three students have been recruited. Other schemes to support medical students include RCPsych awards, regional award schemes, and prizes offered by special interest groups.

Careers Guidance and Information

Every year, the College responds to more than 450 individual queries, sends career materials to around 100 events, and attends careers fairs locally and nationally – including BMJ Careers, Medlink, and the Royal Society of Medicine's Careers Day – reaching around 2,500 people and many more via the College Divisions and Devolved Nations. We encourage all medical schools to engage with RCPsych to ensure they receive support in providing up-to-date and inspiring career advice to their students.

The RCPsych Undergraduate Education Forum

The RCPsych Undergraduate Education Forum was established to bring together the undergraduate teaching leads in psychiatry from each UK medical school. It promotes discussion of core material for undergraduate teaching and enables sharing of best practice. The Forum wants to ensure that interested medical students find it easy to contact someone within their local university department who can provide them with advice and/or signpost them to an appropriate supervisor.

Medical Student Psychotherapy Schemes and Balint Groups

The College aims to make Medical Student Psychotherapy schemes and Balint groups accessible in all medical schools. Balint groups provide a safe space for students to discuss their emotional reactions to their patients' experiences, helping them develop empathy and their capacity to cope with emotional stress. Psychotherapy schemes allow students to learn the core concept of psychotherapy and to practise clinical skills. According to Yakeley et al. (2004), projects which involve medical students offering psychodynamic therapy to a carefully selected patient in an outpatient setting for one session a week for a year have contributed to increases in recruitment to psychiatry.

Conclusion

The support described in this chapter has proved extremely popular. PEEP, 'Extreme Psychiatry', and Pitstop are over-subscribed and students want them to be more accessible. The bigger ambition is to reach a younger audience by raising awareness of psychiatry at all levels of education, including at primary and secondary school levels. Initiatives have already been developed, such as 'I'm a Medic, Get Me Out of Here!', an online outreach programme aimed at informing schoolchildren in England about a particular career in the NHS and trialled in psychiatry for the first time in 2019 (Halder and Mulliez, 2021).

As more people are speaking out about mental illness, we need to open up psychiatry to as many young people as we can – whatever career they end up choosing. With limited resources available, this represents a challenge for everyone involved, and will only be achieved through collaborative effort.

References

Halder, N. and Mulliez, Z. (2021). Encouraging recruitment into psychiatry: Practical initiatives. *BJPsych Bulletin*. **45** (1): 15–22. https://doi.org/10.1192/bjb.2020.53.

Health Education England. (2020). Specialty recruitment: round 1 – acceptance and fill rate. Available from: www.hee.nhs.uk/our-work/medical-recruitment/specialty-recruitment-round-1-acceptance-fill-rate.

Mulliez, Z. (2019). Choose Psychiatry: Guidance for Medical Schools. The Royal College of

Psychiatrists. Available at: www.rcpsych.ac.uk/docs/default-source/become-a-psychiatrist/guidance-for-medical-schools-pdf.pdf?sfvrsn=20f46cae_14

Yakeley, J., Shoenberg, P., and Heady, A. (2004). Who wants to do psychiatry?: The influence of a student psychotherapy scheme – a 10-year retrospective study. *Psychiatric Bulletin*, **28** (6): 208–12. https://doi.org/10.1192/pb.28.6.208.

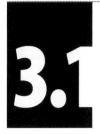

Clinical Placements: Organisation and Supervision

Dr Rekha Hegde

Supervision of a Medical Student

Introduction and the Apprenticeship Model

Most medical students still have the experience of busy, acute hospital posts where people don't know their names and where teaching is done in large groups. Thus, the apprenticeship model we are used to in psychiatry will be a new experience for them and can be a powerful tool for us to show our specialty in a positive light and recruit more trainees into Psychiatry. There is evidence that enthusiastic, interested supervisors make a lasting impression on medical students and trainees, and this can make the difference between a medical student choosing a specialty or not (Passi, 2013). Having a positive role model enables a student to observe and emulate desirable non-clinical skills and attitudes found in the formal, informal, and hidden curriculum (Hafferty, 1998).

For most medical students, the amount of supervision and feedback they receive in a psychiatry placement may be greater than that for other placements. In psychiatry we are used to a variety of types of supervision: clinical supervision, educational supervision, and psychiatric supervision. The supervision of a medical student will encompass aspects of all three kinds of supervision, depending on the situation.

As you will be aware, clinical supervision is related to a clinical interaction such as taking a history or taking blood. Clinical supervision is ideally provided as close as possible to the clinical encounter and will encompass elements of feedback. Educational supervision is about how the student is progressing over the course of their placement and the progress they are making with their education aims and objectives. Both of these are qualitatively different to psychiatric supervision, which as psychiatrists we are familiar with. Psychiatric supervision can be many things, but in its essence is a safe reflective space to process dynamic aspects of therapeutic relationships, maintain professional boundaries, and support development of resilience, well-being, and leadership.

Before the Student Arrives

When you first become a medical-student supervisor you should be sent a pack by the undergraduate medical student lead, which will outline the student's curriculum and the objectives to be met in the post. Many universities offer hybrid posts wherein a student will be in clinical placement for a few days a week with some fixed teaching or simulation slots during the week. You may find that you only see your student for two to three days out of five. Other models for the psychiatric placement may exist; information regarding this should be available from the university.

Before you meet your student, you should clarify with the local undergraduate tutor what the local process is for addressing concerns and familiarise yourself with the undergraduate policy and contact person if concerned. Signs that a student may be struggling are: they don't arrive for the start of their placement, are regularly or persistently absent, cease attending, or exhibit poor time keeping.

Some preparation will make the experience of having a medical student rewarding for yourself and more useful and enjoyable for the student. It is important that you feel you have adequate time in your job plan and that this important educational activity is recognised in job planning and reflected in your Supporting Professional Activity time.

Psychiatry is one of the few community specialties, and it is worth bearing in mind that the student will primarily have had exposure to hospital medicine and acute sites, so working off site in a resource centre may pose a challenge. It is helpful to create a welcome guide to your post, including travel instructions, parking advice, where to get lunch, and how to organise security passes if required in advance. Ideally, the undergraduate lead will have been told in advance if the student can drive or not, as this can be one of the biggest stumbling blocks for a successful psychiatry placement. Medical students are used to being based on one site so some thought needs to be given to how much travelling they have to do and have many sites they would be in on one day.

Having a well-organised placement speaks volumes and makes the student feel that they are valued and included, rather than a nuisance or a hindrance. Medical students can often feel faceless and adrift, so the fact that we have taken the time to get to know them as people, even just knowing their names, may set us apart from other placements in a positive sense. Making them feel part of the team and giving them small, manageable tasks makes them feel as if they are contributing and not merely observing. It is also helpful to explain the relevance of what they are learning for any future career path they might choose; translatability is a powerful motivator for learning. In addition, the GMC states that all newly qualified doctors must be able to safely and sensitively undertake a mental and cognitive state examination, including establishing if the patient is a risk to themselves or others, seeking support, and making referrals if necessary.

You should construct a timetable so that you and your student know where each of you is each day of the week. Ideally this should be sent out a week in advance of your student starting. It is also helpful to have a collection of clinical guides, either on email or as books, that you can send out in advance so they can do some preparation before they arrive (e.g. history-taking, mental state, formulation, risk assessment). The timetable would ideally have slots with different members of the multidisciplinary team, such as psychologists, nursing staff, and occupational therapists, but medical students may prefer to have exposure to a senior medic. A careful balance needs to be sought so the trainee doesn't feel foisted onto non-medical staff because the medical staff are too busy. Medical students also benefit from seeing patients in a variety of settings, such as at home or in a care home, as this is not an experience offered by many other specialties.

Although society is becoming more comfortable with talking about mental health issues in general, it is important to explore any concerns about safety or preconceptions the student may have about psychiatry. Unfortunately, many universities do not feature psychiatry prominently in the undergraduate curriculum and students can often arrive with misconceptions. It is an unfortunate reality that specialty bashing is prevalent, and you may have some work to do in challenging negative stereotypes.

Utilising a variety of teaching formats can be stimulating and promote learning; online videos and recordings of actor consultations can lend themselves well to discussion and are more likely to be remembered by the student. It is also useful to have these as a fall-back should you be called away to an urgent situation or if there are lots of DNAs (Did Not Attend) at an outpatient clinic. Most medical students have theoretical knowledge but require help with honing their communication skills. There are many ways of learning: didactic, experiential, and modelling. At university, students use a mixture of didactic and problem-based learning. In postgraduate medicine experiential learning forms the majority of the learning, but modelling is also an effective and efficient way of teaching, particularly for the subtler non-clinical skills of leadership and time management (hidden and informal curricula). For most medical students knowing how to ask questions and finding a form of words that they are comfortable with can be the hardest part, and role play can be useful in helping them practice this.

The First Meeting

At the first meeting it is useful to discuss aims and objectives, assessments, timetables, and your expectations regarding timekeeping and communication. Most students will have smartphones, so email or text are the preferred methods. You should clarify whom to call in case of an emergency or if they are unwell, and reporting instructions if they are ill. Personal safety is important and should be discussed, and the procedures for wards and visits should be explained.

It is also helpful to have a bank of Royal College of Psychiatrists 'Choose Psychiatry' related information to hand for those medical students who are interested in training to be a psychiatrist; as well as directing them to the local PsychSoc (undergraduate psychiatry society) or giving them information about becoming a student associate of the College. Chapter 2.6 has further information on supporting the psychiatrists of tomorrow.

Professionalism Concerns

All students must adhere to a student agreement, and for medical students this is based on the GMC's guidance, 'Medical Students: Professional Values and Fitness to Practise'. If you have concerns, it is important to raise these with the undergraduate lead and university contact as these issues can resurface throughout a person's career. Early identification can mean that appropriate supports can be put in place. Raising a concern does not automatically lead to a fitness to practise investigation, but allows support to be put into place and monitored.

Box 3.1.1 provides some good practice points when supervising a student in difficulty.

Assessments and Feedback

It is useful to bear in mind that a medical student placement is much shorter than the four- and six-month rotations that doctors in training will have in your team, and that this will have an impact on the dynamics of the student–supervisor relationship. This is most apparent when giving feedback. Feedback must be considered as a supportive, sequential process, rather than a series of unrelated events (Archer, 2006). Thus, in a short placement the trust that develops in a longer attachment will not have time to develop and this can make feedback (particularly negative feedback) harder to give. Again, it is useful to manage

Box 3.1.1 Good Practice Points When Supervising a Student in Difficulty

- Most if not all students will have an advisor of studies and it can be helpful to have permission to contact this person if you have concerns or if the student is struggling.
- It is best to have this conversation at the first meeting so consent is gained and systems are in place should they be needed.
- You should also inform them that you have an obligation to share any concerns with their advisor of studies.
- If you have concerns about a student's performance it is a good idea to make a record of your discussion in a factual and objective manner, ask the student to read and co-sign it, and email a copy as a record of your discussion.

expectations regarding feedback at the first meeting: clarify when and how feedback will be given, how the student feels they respond to feedback, and what its purpose is (i.e. not to criticise but to provide ways of making the execution of a task better/more effective). It is also important to be mindful of how the student might respond to feedback and adjust your language accordingly. The purpose of feedback is to promote self-regulation in students through helping them to recognise any discrepancies between what they are doing and what they ought to do (Nicol, 2006).

Lived Experience

Gordon Johnston

Consideration should also be given to the best manner of ensuring patient views form part of the assessment and feedback process. Where students are directly interacting with patients as part of their placement, this feedback can add another dimension to their learning experience, enhancing reflective thinking and enabling the student to consider how their practice impacts directly on their patients.

Some patients may not wish to provide input, but others will become engaged and can offer a useful insight into particular aspects of the student's practice, such as attitude, communication skills, listening skills, and the ability to form a therapeutic relationship. Presenting this feedback to the student can increase the value of the experience and enable deeper reflection on their emerging practical skills.

Feedback is one of the most important tools in learning (see Box 3.1.2).

There is no benefit to only providing criticism without suggestions for improvement. These suggestions could be used to form a personal development plan with SMART (Specific, Measureable, Achievable, Realistic, Time-measured) objectives. There is evidence that poorly delivered feedback can have a negative effect on learning, well-being, and motivation (Bienstock, 2007).

There are several ways of giving feedback, the most common of which is called Pendleton's rules: both parties state what went well and what did not go so well, and then agree on a plan for improvement, with the student always speaking first.

> **Box 3.1.2 Characteristics of Good Feedback**
>
> Ideally, feedback should:
>
> - be given as soon as possible after the event has been observed;
> - be done in private and be based on observation;
> - be non-judgemental and specific;
> - focus on behaviours;
> - elicit thoughts and feelings; and
> - most importantly, include suggestions for improvement.

The SHARP method was developed for use in clinical simulation and uses Socratic questioning to guide the learner to analyse their performance in a critical way.

Set learning objectives beforehand:

- What would you like to get out of this case?
- How did it go? What went well? Why?
- Address concerns: What did not go so well? Why?
- Review learning points: Were your learning objectives met for this case?
- What did you learn about your clinical, technical, and teamwork skills?
- Plan ahead: What actions can you take to improve your future practice?

Feedback goes both ways and it is important to gain feedback about your post in terms of organisation, content, supervision, and teaching. This can be uploaded to your appraisal account as evidence for recognition of training.

References

Archer, J. C. (2010). State of the science in health professional education: Effective feedback. *Med Educ.* **44** (1): 101–8.

Bienstock, J. L., Katz, N. T., Cox, S. M., Hueppchen, N., and Erickson, S. To the point: medical education reviews – providing feedback. *Am J Obstet Gynaecol.* 2007; **196** (6): 508–51.

Hafferty, F. W. (1998). Beyond curriculum reform: Confronting medicine's hidden curriculum. *Acad Med 1998*; **73** (4): 403–7.

Nicol, D. J. and Macfarlane-Dick, D. (2006). Formative assessment and self-regulated learning: A model and seven principles of good feedback practice. *Studies in Higher Education*; **31**: 199–218.

Passi, V., Johnson, S., Peile, E., Wright, S., Hafferty, F., and Johnson, N. (2013). Doctor role modelling in medical education: BEME Guide No. 27, *Medical Teacher*, **35** (9): e1422–e1436, https://doi.org/10.3109/0142159X .2013.806982.

Teaching and Learning in Clinical Settings

3.2

Dr Amy Manley

"Let the young know they will never find a more interesting,
more instructive book than the patient himself."
Giorgio Baglivi (1669–1707)

The workplace is unlike any other learning setting at medical school. A wealth of learning opportunities with patients at their centre exists for students, though these are neither directly controlled by the teacher nor do they neatly fit within planned learning objectives. Learning is student led, with multiple staff and patients willingly taking on the 'teacher' role despite their primary purpose being to meet a clinical need. An influential portion of learning is unconscious, with far reaching effects on attitudes, reasoning, and professionalism. More than any other setting, the workplace influences the doctor that the student will become. This chapter discusses how to make the most of clinical opportunities to help your students learn effectively without placing an excessive burden on yourself and the team.

Patients at the Centre of Clinical Learning

Seeing patients is why students choose to study medicine, and there is no higher-fidelity place to do this than the workplace. Therefore, focus your student contact time on the clinical application of learning. Placing patients at the heart of every learning experience aids student retention and demonstrates direct relevance to practice. Patients are huge sources of lived experience, so empower them to share this with students (see Figure 3.2.1).

> Top Tip 1 – Hang all teaching on a clinical encounter. If you find yourself imparting free-floating knowledge, consider whether you could direct students to an alternative resource (textbook or website) then catch up with them to apply what they have discovered. You're busy – save your time for the clinical teaching; introduce students to the wealth of learning resources out there.
>
> Top Tip 2 – Consider asking patients for feedback on students. Although this is usually very generous, it can help pick up concerns, particularly with professional behaviour (Reinders et al., 2008).

Consent, Capacity, and Coercion

Most patients retain capacity to consent to student involvement in their care. However, there is a risk of coercion, for example when patients are detained under the Mental Health

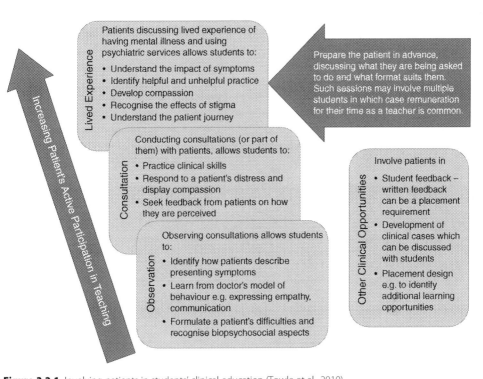

Figure 3.2.1 Involving patients in students' clinical education (Towle et al., 2010).

Act. A lack of capacity does not prohibit student contact, which can be mutually beneficial, but consideration of the patient's expressed wishes and speaking with a carer, relative, or friend, as with any best-interests decision, can be informative.

Top Tip 3 – Support the patient to make an informed decision about seeing students:

- Inform the patient that it is optional and won't affect care
- Consider who should seek consent and do so in advance
- Remind students to introduce themselves and explain the bounds of confidentiality
- Consider documenting the patient's preference for future meetings
- Confirm consent at the time of the meeting
- Additional measures may need to be taken to protect confidentiality (e.g. when seeing a fellow student)

Safety

Students are sometimes unaware of or downplay areas of incompetence, posing a risk to patients. Therefore, ensure adequate supervision with early observation of a student's clinical practice, feedback, team discussion, and clear pathways for escalating issues.

Mental health placements are associated with poorer sense of psychological safety and student satisfaction than placements in physical health settings (Torralba et al., 2016), perhaps due to stigma, unfamiliar environments, younger (more relatable) patient age group, and exposure to emotionally distressing patient accounts. Perceptions of safety can be paradoxically worsened by safety procedures (e.g. wearing an alarm). Therefore, use the 'safety talk' for broader discussion around misperceptions of violence. Psychological safety is enhanced by environments where continuous development is modelled, clinical teachers are cast as allies as opposed to assessors, and open candid discussion is encouraged but confidentiality respected (Johnson et al., 2020).

Top Tip 4 – To contain anxiety and review a student's practice, ensure students know how to access you or another team member to debrief after seeing a patient.

Planned Learning in the Clinical Environment

Clinical learning experiences cannot be standardised without losing the essence of the workplace. However feedback, student activity, and embedding the student as part of the team are helpful and can be planned for. In fact studies consistently suggest that enthusiastic clinical teachers who communicate with and actively involve students are more beneficial to student perceptions of the placement than scheduled teaching time or exposure to specific clinical presentations (Johnson et al., 2020; Sutkin et al., 2008). As long as high-quality learning experiences are provided, variety of experience is an asset for our future workforce.

Active Learning

Keep students active, even when observing, by asking them to complete relevant tasks tailored to their pre-existing knowledge or skill. Tasks may relate to the whole process of patient contact: from information finding, to the more subtle cognitive mechanisms underpinning clinical reasoning, to developing a management plan (see Table A3.2.1 in the Appendix for suggestions to encourage active learning in the workplace).

Top Tip 5 – Ensure students are ACTIVE and ATTENDING to their learning opportunity by setting tasks such as documenting history/mental state examination (MSE), observing question types (e.g. open to closed question ratio and purpose), justifying differential diagnoses, or asking them to offer specific feedback on your performance (this also models a desire for self-development).

Top Tip 6 – Direct students on how to prepare for a task prior to a consultation. This need not take long, but can ensure students have adequate understanding (e.g. 'read pages 20–21 on the mental state examination whilst I review the patient's notes').

Feedback

Feedback and facilitated reflection turn clinical encounters into educational experiences (Eraut, 2000). Opportunities to 'practice psychiatry' and get feedback increase the likelihood of choosing a psychiatric career, whereas patient contact alone does not (Budd et al., 2011).

Valid, reliable feedback is supported by strong teacher–student or team–student relationships. Team discussion and clarity about expectations can also empower the multidisciplinary team to provide meaningful feedback.

> Top Tip 7 – Ensure students get brief feedback on each task or clinical encounter either from you or a colleague. Although time consuming, feedback allows students to quickly become an asset to the team, and contribute to clinical work.

Sequencing and Preparation for Learning

Sequencing learning refers to ordering a student's learning by difficulty so that they are working toward tasks just beyond their current competence. This allows them to add new learning to existing schema, making learning easier. Attending to the complexity and setting of the task, and ensuring that students have an appreciation of the whole task before breaking it into manageable chunks, enables sequencing to occur even with complex patients in an unpredictable clinical environment.

As students transition from observing to observed independent assessments, continue to encourage them to prepare in advance and prime them with key pointers for the consultation (to a maximum of three). Discussing how the student should signal that they have finished when conducting an (or part of an) assessment can also reduce uncertainty (e.g. 'I think that is everything I wanted to ask; Dr Jones, do you have anything you would like to discuss further?'). The Cognitive Apprenticeship Model (Collins and Kapur, 2014) emphasises the changing role of the trainer in supporting a student at different levels of competence, as shown in Figure 3.2.2.

> Top Tip 8 – Ensure that students are supported to work just beyond what they can already do. Get to know their competency level early and discuss their learning needs with other members of the team.
>
> Top Tip 9 – Encourage students to conduct sections of the consultation (e.g. screening for depression) allowing them to practice novel, targeted skills while not becoming overwhelmed by the task.

Developing Clinical Reasoning

Clinical reasoning involves the weighing of information about the patient with pre-existing clinical knowledge to determine what to do next, make diagnoses, devise management plans, and assess risk (Turpin and Higgs, 2017). However it is poorly verbalised by experts, in whom such reasoning largely occurs automatically. This can leave a student wondering how you reached a clinical decision.

Clinical reasoning skills can be developed through:

- Deconstructing and verbalising your reasoning for diagnoses/medication choices/ management strategies (Pinnock et al., 2015).

- Encouraging students to explore the relationship between symptom and diagnosis during a consultation (Dumas et al., 2018) by:
  - 'Ticking off' symptoms on a checklist.
  - Comparing symptoms of two illnesses (e.g. bipolar and schizophrenia).
  - Identifying contrary symptoms which don't fit with the diagnosis.
- Asking the student to express their reasoning for diagnoses and clinical decisions. Socratic questioning can aid discussion (e.g. why do you think this patient is depressed?).
- Discussing diagnosis or diagnostic uncertainty with a patient, with a student observer.
- When presenting a patient's background prior to a consultation, give a brief summary and ask the students what more information they want to know to reach a diagnosis.

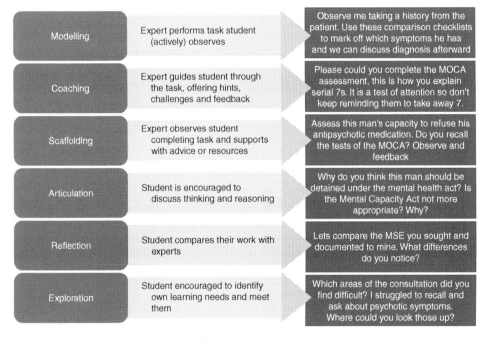

Figure 3.2.2 Cognitive Apprenticeship Model Teaching Methods and their application to a complex patient case (Collins and Kapur 2014).

Structured Presentations

Students need to practice independently, but preparation and debrief are still important. Therefore, consider how this will be done, whether one-to-one or as a group. Structuring a case presentation saves time and enhances learning. One Minute Preceptor (OMP) and Summarise, Narrow, Analyse, Probe, Plan, Select (SNAPPS) (see Table 3.2.1) are structures intended to encourage concise summaries, student reasoning, and targeted teaching. Some universities use a specific format for case presentations across the curriculum. If you, or the student, are not familiar with them, a small amount of training will be needed.

Table 3.2.1 Strategies for case presentations

SNAPPS (Wolpaw et al., 2003)	One Minute Preceptor (OMP) (Neher et al., 1992)
Summarise: Student summarises history, examination, investigations concisely	(1) Commit: Student commits to a most-likely diagnosis
Narrow: Student narrows diagnostic possibilities, identifying 2–3 most likely differentials	(2) Probe: Student justifies the diagnosis with supporting (and contrary) evidence
Analyse: Student analyses differentials, weighing the likelihood and verbalising reasoning	(3) Teach: Clinician discusses a generalisable rule of relevance to the case
Probe: Clinician asks student about areas of uncertainty or difficulty	(4) Praise: Clinician feedback on what was done well
Plan: Plan management for the patient's medical issues	(5) Correct: Clinician feedback on errors made and student and clinician agree next steps to further learning
Select: Select a learning need from the case for student self-study; topics which reflect a generalisable principle are best	

Top Tip 10 – Explain to the student what is expected of them when presenting. Setting time targets can encourage the student to be concise, to recognise key information, and can reduce time pressures (e.g. describe the key points of the patient's history at ward round in under two minutes).

Top Tip 11 – Case discussion groups can be helpful to enable students to learn from each other's case presentations and related discussion, and allow you to teach multiple students together.

Managing Downtime

Inevitably during a student placement there will be downtime (e.g. when a patient declines to see a student). It is useful to have a back-up strategy to keep the student occupied, for example: preparing for the next consultation by reading around the diagnosis, summarising patient notes, or seeking collateral information from the care-coordinator; debriefing from the last consultation by developing a list of differential diagnoses; signposting relevant resources to address learning needs already identified; or having case examples or clinical reasoning exercises which the student can work through.

Top Tip 12 – Ask students to keep a log of learning objectives/questions from discussions and debriefs. They can then use downtime to look these topics up.

The Team in Teaching

You are likely to host a student as part of a wider multidisciplinary team. This enriches the student experience, encourages understanding and respect of different clinical roles, and enables exposure to a breadth of clinical practices and teaching styles. It can impact on the team, particularly when placements are brief so there is little opportunity to see improvement, turnover is high, or students are unprofessional and demanding. It is therefore essential to involve the multidisciplinary team (MDT) when planning to host students, to identify how they would like to be involved, and to assess the impact of hosting students on the team. Remember to consider all the students your team supports, not only medical students, and how you and the team can support the learning of them all. Hosting students from multiple disciplines is an excellent opportunity for facilitating interprofessional learning. If you need more 'carrot' then investigate the teaching CPD (Continuing Professional Development) or training requirements of colleagues, and whether a portion of the income generated by your NHS trust for hosting students could be sent directly to support your team in their educational roles.

Tacit Knowledge and Unconscious Learning

Although this chapter has primarily focussed on the explicit learning experiences available in the workplace, the majority of learning occurs unconsciously. Unconsciously acquired tacit knowledge enhances our psychiatric practice, guiding our professional identity and approach to patients and making it possible to perform tasks more quickly; however, it is also a source of bias and stigma. Therefore, as a clinical teacher, it is essential that we attend to the learning environment, because role models, professional behaviour, team dynamics, the student's role in the team, and other environmental factors (e.g. where students sit) all tell the student what it means to be a psychiatrist. Discussion and reflection with the student on placement experiences, particularly those which are emotionally charged or potentially negative, can make unconscious learning conscious so it can be examined. This allows misconceptions to be addressed and allows us to steer the tacit knowledge acquired by students, thereby reducing misconceptions about our work. In turn, this will encourage a compassionate and competent approach to patients with mental health problems and reduce stigma, encouraging parity of esteem and increasing the likelihood students will choose psychiatry as a career. Cruess et al. (2015) emphasise the value of workplace socialisation to professional learning, and suggestions for supporting this process as mapped to their model are shown in Figure 3.2.3.

> Top Tip 13 – Attend to the environment: Where are the students? Do they have space? Do they have access to the facilities? Are they sitting at the table or are they at the back? Do people engage them in clinical work? Are people providing professional role models?
>
> Top Tip 14 – When students experience events which are emotionally charged or personally significant, take the time to discuss and reflect together. Understanding their experience of the situation will allow misperceptions to be addressed and reinforce learning.

Summary

In the workplace, effective learning opportunities have patients at their centre. Save time by signposting resources which students can use to address learning needs so you can focus your student contact time on clinically meaningful tasks. Whether students are observing you, or working independently, prime them beforehand; ensure they are active during the

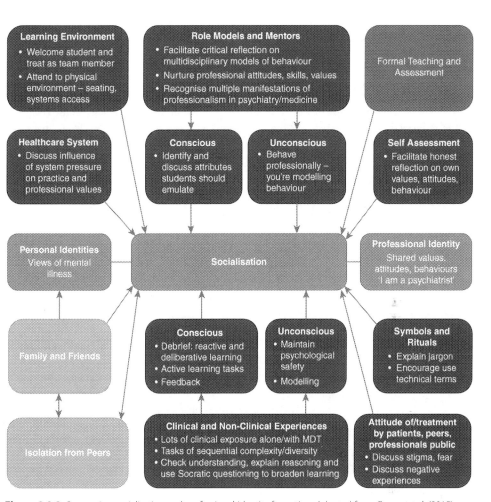

Figure 3.2.3 Supporting socialisation and professional identity formation. Adapted from Cruess et al. (2015)

clinical encounter, and provide feedback afterwards. Sequencing clinical tasks, verbalising reasoning, and use of case presentation models aid understanding and identification of learning needs. Finally, remember that much of the learning in the workplace occurs unconsciously, therefore role modelling and reflective discussions are important to guide attitude and value development.

References

Budd, S., Kelley, R., Day, R., Variend, H., and Dogra, N. (2011). Student attitudes to psychiatry and their clinical placements. *Med Teach.* **33** (11): e586–92.

Collins, A. and Kapur, M. (2014). Cognitive Apprenticeship. In R. K. Sawyer (ed.), *The Cambridge Handbook of the Learning Sciences*, pp. 47–60. Cambridge University Press.

Cruess, R. L., Cruess, S. R., Boudreau, J. D., Snell, L., and Steinert, Y. (2015). A schematic representation of the professional identity formation and socialization of medical students and residents: a guide for medical educators. *Acad Med.* **90** (6): 718–25.

Dumas, D., Torre, D. M., and Durning, S. J. (2018). Using Relational Reasoning Strategies to Help Improve Clinical Reasoning Practice. *Acad Med.* **93** (5). Available at: https://journals.lww.com/ academicmedicine/Fulltext/2018/05000/ Using_Relational_Reasoning_Strategies_ to_Help.29.aspx

Eraut, M. (2000). Non-formal learning and tacit knowledge in professional work. *Br J Educ Psychol.* **70** (1): 113–36.

Johnson, C. E., Keating, J. L., and Molloy, E. K. (2020). Psychological safety in feedback: What does it look like and how can educators work with learners to foster it? *Med Educ.* **54** (6): 559–70.

McGee, S. R. and Irby, D. M. (1997). Teaching in the outpatient clinic. Practical tips. *J Gen Intern Med.* Apr; **12** Suppl 2\ (Suppl 2): S34–40. Available from: https://pubmed .ncbi.nlm.nih.gov/9127242

Neher, J. O., Gordon, K. C., Meyer, B., and Stevens, N. (1992). A five-step 'microskills' model of clinical teaching. *J Am Board Fam Pract.* **5** (4): 419–24.

Pinnock, R., Young, L., Spence, F., Henning, M., and Hazell, W. (2015). Can think aloud be used to teach and assess clinical reasoning in graduate medical education? *J Grad Med Educ.* Sep; **7** (3): 334–7. Available from: https://pubmed.ncbi.nlm.nih.gov/26457135

Reinders, M. E., Blankenstein, A. H., van Marwijk, H. W. J., Schleypen, H.,

Schoonheim, P. L., and Stalman, W. A. B. (2008). Development and feasibility of a patient feedback programme to improve consultation skills in general practice training. *Patient Educ Couns.* **72** (1): 12–9.

Sutkin, G., Wagner, E., Harris, I., and Schiffer, R. (2008). What makes a good clinical teacher in medicine? A review of the literature. *Acad Med.* **83** (5). Available from: https://journals .lww.com/academicmedicine/Fulltext/2008/ 05000/What_Makes_a_Good_Clinical_ Teacher_in_Medicine__A.7.aspx

Torralba, K. D., Loo, L. K., Byrne, J. M., et al. (2016). Does Psychological Safety Impact the Clinical Learning Environment for Resident Physicians? Results From the VA's Learners' Perceptions Survey. *J Grad Med Educ.* Dec; **8** (5): 699–707. Available from: https://pubmed .ncbi.nlm.nih.gov/28018534

Towle, A., Bainbridge, L., Godolphin, W., et al. (2010). Active patient involvement in the education of health professionals. *Med Educ.* **44** (1): 64–74.

Turpin, M. and Higgs, J. (2017). Clinical reasoning and evidence-based practice. In T. Hoffmann, S. Bennett, and C. B. Del Mar (eds.) *Evidence-Based Practice Across the Health Professions*, pp. 364–83. Elsevier.

Wolpaw, T. M., Wolpaw, D. R., and Papp, K. K. (2003). SNAPPS: A learner-centered model for outpatient education. *Acad Med.* **78** (9). Available from: https://journals.lww.com/ academicmedicine/Fulltext/2003/09000/ SNAPPS__A_Learner_centered_Model_for_ Outpatient.10.aspx

Appendix

Suggested activities to encourage active learning

Novice Student	More Experienced Student
Seeing a patient together	
Knowledge and skills:	**Putting it all together:**
• Document the MSE or history (following a certain structure)	• Review the patients notes and give a 2-minute summary. This may focus on a specific aspect, e.g. progress since last appointment, treatment history, clinical features on previous presentations
• Identify at least 3 additional questions you would like to ask the patient	
Reasoning:	• Complete focussed part of the consultation which may involve:
• List presenting symptoms as to how they fit with top differentials (student has sheet with columns for the two diagnoses, neither and both), to document symptoms as they arise	• Eliciting information e.g. screen for symptoms such as psychotic phenomena, assess and mitigate risk of further self harm, complete cognitive assessment
	• Explain diagnosis or medication (e.g. SSRI) when starting, to the patient
Communication:	• Complete the full observed consultation. You can set a focus for feedback (usually something they need to work on) for example:
• Count the types of questions I am using (open, closed, affirmations, reflections, etc.)	• Avoiding closed questions towards the start of consultation (time them!)
• Feedback on my communication skills (at least 3 specific positives and negatives)	• Show empathy
	• Personal history
	• Lead a section of the ward round or meeting e.g. facilitating multidisciplinary discussion
After the consultation	
Debrief / feedback from tasks above	**Debrief / feedback on the tasks above**
Knowledge and skills:	• focussing on key points only to avoid cognitive overload
• Write up the clinical notes / MSE (remember to check them)	**Putting it all together:**
Reasoning:	• Present the patient using an educational structure e.g. SNAPPS/OMP (see main chapter)
• Explain reasoning behind clinical decisions	• Write up a patient formulation
• Identify as many differential diagnoses as possible	• Seek collateral history
	• Liaise with MDT colleagues / patient's GP to plan management

(cont.)

Novice Student	More Experienced Student
Communication:	• Complete tasks relevant to the agreed management plan e.g. phlebotomy, discussing behavioural activation with the patient, looking up medications in the BNF
• <2-minute presentation of the key points from the assessment as if to a ward round. Follow a specific model (e.g. OMP, SNAPPS)	
Independent Activities	
Knowledge and Skills:	**Putting it all together:**
• Elicit a medical history from a patient (something they may have already practised frequently) with a comorbid mental health problem. This can gradually be built upon to include further psychiatric information	• See a patient independently and present their case at the ward round • Write a patient/GP letter • Where diagnostic uncertainty remains, explain what you think are the most likely diagnoses and why
Reasoning:	• Develop a proposed management plan for a patient and describe its pros and cons
• Based on background information, determine likely differential diagnoses, and research them to determine which is most likely	• Conduct a cognitive assessment and interpret findings • Use a psychiatric rating scale • Present a case to another student and discuss an aspect to reach a joint decision about appropriate treatment

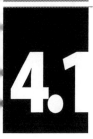

How to Give a Lecture

Professor Nisha Dogra and Dr Sophie Butler

This chapter begins by summarising the reasons lectures continue to have a place in medical education and then considers how a lecturer can prepare and deliver an interactive lecture.

Exercise 1

Think of 'good' and 'bad' lectures you have attended. Reflect on what, from your perspective, made them that way. Now:

1. Make a list of the characteristics of a good lecturer
2. Make a list of the features of a good lecture

Lectures as an Effective Teaching Strategy

There can be a tendency to assume that lectures have little function in education today. However, we believe that they remain an effective teaching tool, if used in the right context and if applied appropriately.

A lecture is a formal presentation to a large audience. Teaching a large group brings unique challenges, not least because lectures often take place in a traditional tiered lecture theatre, which increases the barriers for creating interactions. Nevertheless, it is critical to consider how to incorporate interaction in a lecture because there is evidence that, for most students, it improves learning (Price and Mitchell, 1993). You may worry that interaction costs time and content, but there is a strong argument that a balance can be struck to maximise the effectiveness of the lecture format (Huxham, 2005).

The nature of lecturing has changed with technology. Some students may attend the lecture in person, others may watch a recorded version. Students may prefer recorded versions for convenience or so that they can control their learning, accelerating the speed (up to two and half times normal!). This may speed up knowledge acquisition and help them stay focussed (Cardall et al., 2008). You may even be delivering a lecture completely remotely in the virtual world (as discussed later in this chapter).

Preparing for the Lecture

Effective teaching depends on effective preparation. It is easy for the audience to tell when the lecturer has prepared or not. The less experienced you are the more time preparation takes, but being experienced does not remove the need for preparation.

When you are invited to give a lecture, clarify issues such as the time you have, the audience, and the context. Are the learning outcomes for you to set or are there predefined

---

Box 4.1.1 The Role of Lectures

Lectures are effective when you want to . . ..

- Deliver low-level cognitive skills type learning – that is, giving basic information rather than synthesis or evaluation
- Enable dissemination of information quickly to large audiences
- Provide an overview
- Provide context or framework for other activities (for example, using a lecture to lay the foundation before small group work to build on this learning)
- Arousing student curiosity to motivate greater learning
- Keep relative teacher-led control over the direction of the teaching

Lectures are less effective when you want to . . ..

- Teach psychomotor skills (students need to be able to practice these)
- Teach high-level cognitive skills such as evaluation
- Change student attitudes and or feelings
- Impart detailed information (most of this, if given in a lecture, is unlikely to be retained)

Difficulties with lectures are that . . .

- Communication can be just one way, from teacher to student
- There is little or no feedback regarding the effectiveness of the learning
- Students may take on a passive role and be disengaged

Table generated from Reece and Walker (2000), Minton (1997), and Sullivan and McIntosh (1996).

---

outcomes? Familiarise yourself with students' previous learning associated with the subject and ensure that the lecture is relevant to the audience it is meant for.

Use the lecture as a means of hooking students and encouraging them to learn more rather than a method to cover everything about the subject.

Common sense tells you that no-one, not even the most enthusiastic student, can pay attention for a whole hour. Incorporate 'breaks' every 15–20 minutes to summarise or shake things up with an interactive activity (e.g. an online poll or exercise in pairs). Pausing is an effective way to provide structure and allows students to catch up and refocus.

Introduction

Give students a guide as to what they should expect to learn and signpost as you move from one topic to another. Provide a clear context and be explicit about the relevance of the teaching to their needs. If you plan on revisiting topics, let students know the purpose for including them.

Main Body

Less is more, so avoid giving too much information that students can get from any textbook. Use the contact time to highlight key issues and focus on the principles rather than the detail.

Summary

Recap the main points. Do not introduce new material in the summary.

Questions

Leave time for questions, even if only a few minutes. Before the lecture consider the questions you might ask the audience and questions they might ask you. Be prepared to role model not knowing everything – this is an important lesson in medicine!

Preparing Your Materials
Slides

The purpose of slides is to provide a guide to the audience and an aide-memoir to the lecturer. Using slides can make teaching more accessible to students who may have hearing impairments or find it difficult to remain attentive.

Handouts

Some view it as disadvantageous to give handouts out before the lecture, believing students will then not attend. However, it allows students to prepare and it is useful for students follow the lecture alongside the slides. Some students may just rest easy, but others will be more engaged in the learning knowing they do not have to take notes and they can really listen.

Using Additional Technology

You may want to play videos or use online interactive platforms (e.g. PollEv or Mentimeter). These allow you to create questions or polls that students can answer using their phones or laptops. They can create some really great real-time visuals (e.g. MCQ answers, word clouds, ranking of topics). This can aid interaction and engagement, but you must always prepare the running of this in advance: have the video set up at point ready to play; have the poll integrated into your presentation or ready to go in a browser window. It is essential to have

---

Box 4.1.2 Tips for Better Slides

Tips for better slides

- Keep your slides simple
- Use animation judiciously bearing in mind your skill level and available software
- Use a font that is easily read: fonts like OpenDyslexic and Fs Me have been specifically designed for those with learning difficulties (see Recite Me for more information)
- Be thoughtful in your colour scheme (e.g. use a colour-blindness-friendly palette)
- A font of less than 18 means you have too much on your slide
- Ensure the number of slides fit the time allocated, if you do mistime you can skip over non-essential slides with an apology, but this may suggest poor preparation
- Remember that handouts can be more detailed than your slides

a fall-back option should the technology fail, and be realistic about expectations for yourself. Don't try lots of new things at the same time.

Rehearsing the Lecture

Early in your career and for important lectures, rehearse them – this helps build confidence and provides an opportunity to get feedback from colleagues.

Exercise 2

Imagine you have been asked to give a lecture on 'Suicide Risk Assessment' to Year 3 medical students who are new to this topic.

1. Prepare a session outline with an introduction, main body, and summary.
2. Use one of the above websites to create two interactive activities that you could incorporate into your lecture.

Delivering the Lecture
Before the Lecture

Arrive on time at the very least, but early if you are not familiar with the venue.

It sounds obvious, but make yourself comfortable by going to the bathroom and ensuring you have access to a drink. Distractions may minimise your impact.

Prepare your environment: survey the room and remove any distraction such a previous lesson on whiteboards or flipcharts. Make sure you know how the audio-visuals work.

Delivering the Lecture

Appear confident: as many would say, 'fake it until you make it' – the more you do this, the more comfortable you will be. A nervous or anxious speaker does not inspire confidence. Remember, good lecturers come in all shapes and sizes; students don't need an encyclopaedia recited to them. Try to enjoy exploring your style and what you bring to the table.

Box 4.1.3 Do's and Don'ts for Delivering the Lecture

Do's	Don'ts
✓ Speak with conviction and commitment, it really does matter	✗ Read from notes or read out the slides without expanding as this can be frustrating for the audience and minimises engagement
✓ Speak clearly, without rushing	
✓ Make good eye contact across the room	✗ Try and cover too much – less really is more
✓ Relate the contents of the lecture to the students' needs	
✓ Keep to time	

Introduction to The Lecture

First impressions matter, so the introduction warrants a special mention. Some lecturers use quotes, anecdotes, or jokes to engage with the audience. This is discussed more in the section 'The Use of Self', but be careful with using strategies that are at odds with your personality. The opening minutes can also be used to clarify the students' educational needs. If they have had to undertake some preparation, get feedback to identify what you may need to spend more time on.

Making Lectures Interactive and Engaging

The Use of Self

Verbal communication is clearly vital, but it can be reinforced with effective and positive non-verbal communication. Using eye contact to gauge responses is a useful way of obtaining feedback on whether the lecture is pitched at the right level. Avoid just gazing at one member of the audience – a common trap. Cover all areas of the room and consider how you may be able to physically move around the space to change students' focus.

Humour can be effective, but it is safer not to tell risky jokes. Develop your own style by watching others and using the techniques that fit with your personality. You also have access to a wealth of clinical experience and that is often a great way of engaging students. Using clinical examples and anecdotes brings theory and facts to life and can illustrate key points.

Questions

Questions are an excellent way of engaging others, and time constraints make rhetorical questions especially useful. For example, if wanting to highlight the impact of stigma in mental health you might ask students to consider their own views or how they think the media portrays the issue.

Questions are also useful to check whether students have understood your lecture. Getting students to raise their hands to indicate learning can provide quick and effective feedback. Or, you could pose a question and get students to call out the answers, which you can ask one of them to write up. This makes the teaching more of a shared experience. Questions should not be used to humiliate or embarrass students.

Using Handouts and Interactive Exercises

Handouts can also be a highly effective way of increasing interaction. Activities such as students having to complete lists where a stem is provided or where they must annotate a diagram or fill in missing words may enliven the lecture.

You may adapt and incorporate small group activities: for example, ask them to discuss in pairs for a few minutes or use technology (see section 'Using Additional Technology').

Lived Experience Inputs

Gordon Johnston

Another method of both increasing the effectiveness of a lecture and of retaining audience attention can be to provide additional inputs alongside your own. This can break up the session, as well as introducing a different viewpoint for students to consider.

One option is to invite people with lived experience to deliver talks as part of a lecture. So, for example, a lecture on stigma in society could usefully include input from someone outlining their own experiences of stigma and giving a direct first-person account of how this has impacted on their life. In combination with the theoretical input, this can be a powerful method of reinforcing learning, and can also encourage students to consider the subject under discussion from a different perspective.

When well planned and integrated into the programme, lived experience input can provide additional learning for students and also enhance their understanding of the subject under discussion. This form of learning is generally well received, with positive student feedback and achievement of deeper understanding.

Lived experience input can be achieved by direct delivery or, alternatively, by recording a talk to be played to students during a lecture. This involves additional preparation but creates a resource that can be used multiple times (with appropriate consent, of course).

Remote Lectures

The use of online platforms to deliver lectures is an emerging area of medical education. You cannot simply translate your face-to-face lecture into the virtual world. The first consideration is to be familiar with the technology you are using. You do not need to be an expert, but you need to know what is possible with a given platform in order to use it effectively. For example, depending on what you use, there may be inbuilt functions such as chat functions, screen-sharing, hand raising, breakout rooms, white-board, and polling options.

Some institutions only support a particular platform due to the security offered. If you have the choice then think about how you can optimise security (e.g. password protection, waiting room function, having to sign into registered account). Be explicit about your consent for recording.

To help prepare and deliver your session

- Practice using the platform beforehand and accessing the functions you need.
- Think about your camera angle: no-one wants to see only your eyebrows. Sit so that all of your facial expressions can be seen. If you are someone who expresses themselves through body language, you may want your hands and some of your body in shot.
- Set some ground rules at the beginning; you may want participants to have their microphones muted. Let students know when and how they can ask questions and if you will be monitoring the chat function.
- Consider asking students to turn their videos on so that you can see their responses and react – this helps keep you engaged too! Remember that you can't make eye contact with individuals, but you might have other advantages such as being able to see their names.
- Don't let the virtual world intimidate you into reducing interactivity: be creative.

- Be mindful that not everyone has access to private spaces so if sharing patient stories or covering sensitive topics, you may want to ask students to use headphones if possible.
- Some students may not have the best internet speed; be patient with connectivity issues!

Developing as a Lecturer

We all teach differently and have different strengths, so this chapter can only provide a general guide. It is essential that you adopt a reflective stance and get as much feedback as possible from students, peers, and mentors. If your lecture has been recorded, you have the uncomfortable (!) but valuable opportunity to watch yourself and learn from it. Lecturing is a skill, and like any skill you can improve it through practice and active development.

Box 4.1.4 10 Key Points for Delivering a Lecture

1. Remember that the lecture enables the delivery of key principles and the opportunity to provide an overview to a large audience.
2. When agreeing to a lecture, establish who is it for and the context.
3. Be clear about learners' needs and connect your lecture to their existing knowledge.
4. Have a clear and logical structure that you share with the audience.
5. Don't try to cover too much – less is more.
6. Numbers may make it difficult to engage with the audience so use a variety of techniques to increase audience participation (e.g. questions, buzz groups, interactive handouts, online platforms).
7. If you are using technology, familiarise yourself with it beforehand and have a back-up plan for if it fails.
8. Keep the audience thinking and, where possible, ask challenging questions, even if they are rhetorical.
9. Remember to have a beginning (tell them what you are going to tell them), a middle (tell them what you want to tell them) and an ending (tell them what you have told them)
10. Always leave adequate time for a summary and questions.

References

Cardall, S., Krupat, E., and Ulrich, M. (2008). Live lectures versus video-recorded lectures: Are students voting with their feet. *Academic Medicine*, **83**; 12: 1174–8.

Huxham, M. (2005). Learning in lectures: Do interactive windows help? *Active Learning in Higher Education*, **6**; 1: 17–31.

Mentimeter. (n.d.). Available at: www .mentimeter.com/ (accessed 26 March 2022).

Microsoft. (n.d.). Make your powerpoint presentation presentations accessible to people with disabilities. Available at: https://support.microsoft.com/en-us/office/make-your-powerpoint-presentations-accessible-to-people-with-disabilities-6f7772 b2-2f33-4bd2-8ca7-dae3b2b3ef25#:~:text= Use%20the%20Accessibility%20Checker%20 and,in%20the%20Reading%20Order% 20pane (accessed 26 March 2022).

Minton, D. (1997). *Teaching Skills in Further and Adult Education*. Revised 2nd Ed. Basingstoke: MacMillan Press Limited.

Pollev. (n.d.). *PollEv*. Available at: https://pollev .com/home (accessed 26 March 2022).

Price, D. A. and Mitchell, C. A. (1993). A model for clinical teaching and learning. *Medical Education*, **27**; **1**: 62–8.

Recite Me. (n.d.). Accessible Font Guide. Available at: https://reciteme.com/uploads/ articles/accessible_fonts_guide.pdf (accessed 12 August 2020).

Reece, I. and Walker, S. (2000). *A Practical Guide to Teaching, Training and Learning*. 4th ed. Tyne and Wear: Business Education Publishers Limited.

Sullivan, R. and McIntosh, N. (1996). Delivering Effective Lectures. JHPIEGO Strategy Paper accessed on 19 April 2009 at: http://www .reproline.jhu.edu/english/6read/6training/ lecture/delivering_lecture.htm.

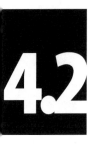

How to Do Small Group Teaching

Professor Nisha Dogra and Dr Khalid Karim

Introduction

Small group teaching can seem challenging, with numerous potential pitfalls. In this chapter we will look at the strengths and challenges of this mode of teaching and provide practical tips to improve the learning environment.

What is Small Group Teaching?

Small group teaching can be defined as teaching that aims to promote student learning through working with peers and a facilitator. The types of small groups that are most common are:

Tutorials – the students are set a task or assignment and the tutor provides support to meet that task with a smaller number of students. In undergraduate teaching this might be used for helping students prepare their clinical portfolios.

Seminars – students research a topic area, then present their findings to their peers, which results in group discussion and further learning. Seminars tend to be led by the learners, but the context and preparation required needs to be clearly identified. An example of this might be the use of antidepressants. To encourage student participation once the student has presented, the others ask questions and share their experience of this medication in practice. The facilitator can clarify and direct the students learning. If students are not experienced their presentations can be lengthy and/or poorly prepared, so the facilitator needs to monitor this carefully. At the end of the seminar the facilitator or a student should summarise the learning.

Discussion groups – the students discuss a specific issue with specific learning tasks: for example, how to manage a disorder or situation. This is a useful format when you want students to explore their own attitudes, but it requires careful and sensitive facilitation. Discussion groups can easily lose focus, and it can be lengthy process to hear all perspectives and allow everyone to have a say.

Workshops – an opportunity to develop skills in a simulated situation and link the theory with practice.

Problem-based learning groups – in problem-based curricula, learning groups are an important method of learning. There are usually some supplementary lectures, but most of the learning is through group work, some of which is facilitated and some of which is student-led and student-managed.

Box 4.2.1 Goals of Small Group Teaching

The goals of small group teaching include:
- Development of higher cognitive understanding by building on key principles
- Development of key competencies
- Development of effective communication skills
- Personal development
- Promotion of student independence
- Development of group management skills

(Entwistle et al., 1992)

When is Small Group Teaching Appropriate?

The primary purpose of small group teaching is not to impart facts, key concepts, or principles, but to help students reinforce their learning by analysing, evaluating, and critiquing their learning and understanding. Small group teaching can also be an excellent opportunity for students to explore their attitudes in a safe environment and practise applying some of their learning.

Small Group Sizes

In 'small' group teaching, the number of participants can vary from 4 to 60! Realistically, the most effective group size is 8–12 students as it prevents the quiet students from 'hiding' but enables the tutor to manage the group and direct the learning. Larger group teaching needs careful planning, and it helps to consider everything that needs to be covered beforehand, dividing the tasks between subgroups of the whole group. This should ensure that students actively listen to each other as they are aware that they are not covering all the material. It also prevents feedback from becoming too repetitive, which may occur if everyone is completing the same task. From experience, no matter how many times you ask the group spokesperson to only add anything new, most will recap the subgroup's whole discussion. Small group teaching is less about size than function.

Strategies for Small Group Teaching

When the small group is not actually that small there are several techniques that can be used to effectively make the working groups smaller. Jaques (2003) and Reece and Walker (2000) provide an overview of the types of strategies that can be used.

Brainstorming

This is a problem-solving technique used to generate a few ideas or solutions very quickly – usually taking just a few minutes. It is often used to quickly generate ideas which can then be further explored. Brainstorming can be a useful warm-up exercise and allows freedom to think outside the box, thereby encouraging creativity.

Group Round (Round Robin)

Each person has a short period of time to say something in turn to the whole group. The direction can be decided by the first speaker or the facilitator. Jaques (2003) suggests that more interest and energy is generated if the first person chooses who should go second, the second chooses who goes third, and so on. This is less likely to be successful in groups that are not familiar with each other.

Buzz Groups

Students are asked to turn to their neighbour and discuss an issue or problem. This is good for ensuring everyone has an opportunity to express an opinion and enables sharing of perspectives that may be difficult with a larger audience. The process is an effective method for developing listening and communication skills as members can be asked to relay back what their partner said.

Snowballing

Snowball groups (sometimes called pyramid groups) are an extension of buzz groups. The discussion work begins in pairs; two pairs then become a four, the four becomes an eight, and then the eight shares to the whole group. In this way the group's learning increases in a staged way. However, the group task needs to be focussed to prevent disarray from the reorganisation. Too much repetition can be avoided by building in layers of complexity as the group size increases.

Fishbowls

The usual configuration has an inner group discussing an issue or topic while the outer group listens with a specific task in mind, for example to identify key themes raised or issues not addressed. If the inner group was role playing, the outer group may provide structured feedback on specific skills, such as communication.

Crossover Groups

Students are divided into subgroups that are then split into different subgroups, and learning from the previous group is shared with the new group to maximise the sharing of information. Keeping tabs on this kind of activity can be difficult if there are many students and the facilities are limited. It can be useful to give students a number or colour and ask certain digits or colours to move to ensure smoother movement between group formations.

Online Groups

Online teaching, including group-based learning for the types of teaching discussed above, is increasingly used, either blended with face-to-face learning or as the main method of delivering education. There are several challenges to delivering groups online, technological issues being a main one, but there can also be encouraging engagement of the group and facilitation of a positive dynamic for learning.

Lived Experience Facilitation

Gordon Johnston

An effective variation on small group teaching is to involve a group of people with lived experience in the facilitation process. For example, an initial presentation to the whole class could be followed by smaller breakout discussions. This is easiest in person but can also be delivered remotely with the correct software.

These small groups allow direct interaction and discussion for a limited period of time, perhaps developing themes or agreeing on key messages from the initial presentation. Outcomes can then be fed back to the whole group, enhancing learning by allowing discussion and revealing contrast between the various small groups' conclusions.

This type of session needs careful planning and timetabling in order to achieve maximum benefit for the students. However, where perhaps three or four facilitators work together as a planning and delivery group, the result can be of great benefit, and tends to achieve excellent feedback from students.

The Role of the Facilitator

The London Deanery (2009) outlines that there are three main tasks that the small group facilitator needs to manage simultaneously:

- The group and the dynamics which occur;
- The activities;
- The learning that takes place.

Preparing for Small Group Teaching

For many small group teachers, the outcomes and contents for the sessions will usually be predefined. However, even if this is the case it is still worth reviewing them with the students to ensure there is a shared understanding and that as a teacher there are no incorrect assumptions about their knowledge base.

Room Layout

Figure 4.2.1 shows the ways that rooms may be set up to ensure maximum student participation. The common factor in all the layouts is that group members face each other, thereby enabling face-to-face interactions. The room set-up is often not within the tutor's control, but whenever possible these types of layouts ought to be secured.

In options 1 and 2, everyone can see each other but there is potential for the focus to be on the teacher. In the other options the teacher is an integral part of the group. Tables can be helpful if students need to write or refer to texts, although some regard them as a physical obstacle and possible barrier. Option 3 may be less useful as the teacher has a better view of some students than others and this can lead to some students being accidentally excluded. Often the person next to us in such a formation is the one we can see least well.

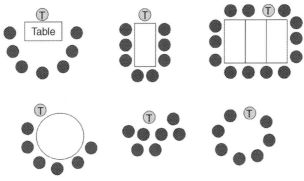

From Jacques (2000)

Figure 4.2.1 Examples of room layouts for small group teaching (from Jaques, 2000).

Box 4.2.2 Rules of Group Working

Commonly accepted rules of group working are:

- Emphasise the need for a safe learning environment
- Show respect for different perspectives
- To listen respectfully, no 'put downs'
- Views to be challenged respectfully
- Everyone needs to do their share and prepare appropriately
- Keep to time
- Leave personal agendas outside the session
- Participants should only share information about themselves that they feel comfortable sharing
- Confidentiality needs to be emphasised, especially if discussing personal or sensitive issues

---

Running the Group

In groups which are familiar with each other only minimal introductions may be required. In other contexts (e.g. at conferences), introductions can be helpful so that the facilitator better understands the learners' needs, but ensure that a disproportionate amount of time is not spent on introductions. At the outset provide the learning outcomes and an outline of the session plan. When the students are engaged in tasks it is useful for the facilitator to move between groups to help move the discussion, but also to help students stay focussed.

If the group members are familiar with each other, they should be aware of the ground rules for the group, but it may be useful to reiterate them.

Allowing the group to challenge different perspectives is important for effective learning. It is the facilitator's role to ensure that this is done respectfully and professionally. Some issues may evoke strong responses. It is appropriate to allow expression of these if any conflict is resolved – this is an important part of group functioning and learning so should not be avoided if the situation arises.

Potential Problems and How to Address Them

Small group teaching is a rewarding process, but it can pose difficulties. These can broadly be described as goal-based problems, group interaction-based problems, student issues, and tutor issues (after Tiberius, 1999).

Goal Related

Tiberius (2000) identified potential problems with group goals as:

1. Goals are unclear
2. Goals are unattainable
3. Goals are unacceptable

Group Interaction

These problems can be summarised as:

1. Lack of interaction
2. Teacher dominates interaction
3. Students participate unequally

Student Issues

Many of these issues have been incorporated into the previous discussion. Factors which affect student learning in general are also factors which affect small group learning, such as difficulties in their personal lives. Specific problems in this area include:

1. Inadequate preparation by the student
2. Students do not participate, do so grudgingly, or are hostile
3. Some students dominate the session
4. Superficial learning happens
5. Students want certainty and answers rather than to work through the issues

Tutor Issues

The tutor is an essential part of the group process and it is important to recognise the difficulties which can affect this function. The skills needed to run groups are not innate and require development. Issues may include:

1. Inadequate preparation by the tutor
2. Tutor fails to use small group environment effectively
3. Tutor does not engage the students
4. Tutor is overly controlling or fails to control the session
5. Tutor is overly critical
6. Tutor is unaware or fails to acknowledge student responses, especially if difficult issues are raised

Box 4.2.3 Summary of Small Group Teaching

1. Small group teaching is used to get learners to talk, debate, discuss, and engage in problem-solving exercises. It is an opportunity to maximise learner participation.
2. Encourages students to question, criticise, analyse, evaluate, speculate, think, and understand.
3. Set a context and ensure that the discussions are directed towards the achievement of the learning objectives.
4. Make sure the learners know what is expected of them and if they need to prepare anything in advance; ensure they have plenty of notice if so.
5. Be prepared with a range of questions that cover a wide range of cognitive skills, from recall, through application to problem solving.
6. Be prepared to elaborate and rephrase questions if necessary.
7. Ensure an adequate wait time after asking a question and actively listen to the answer.
8. Respond to answers by providing explanations, sensitive feedback on misunderstandings, and praise for understanding.
9. Encourage learners to talk with each other – break the group up into smaller groups if necessary.
10. Ensure the outcome results of the discussions are summarised.
11. Refer to the context of the learning objectives to provide a sense of cohesion, completeness, and achievement.

References

Entwistle, N. J., Thompson, S. and Tait, H. (1992). *Guidelines for Promoting Effective Learning in Higher Education*. Centre for Research and Learning and Information, University of Edinburgh.

Jaques, D. (2000). *Learning in Groups: A Handbook for Improving Group Learning*, 3rd ed. London: Kogan Page.

Jaques, D. (2003). ABC of learning and teaching in medicine: Teaching small groups. *British Medical Journal*, **326**; 7387: 492–4.

London Deanery (2009). Small Group Teaching. Available at: https://london.hee.nhs.uk/fd-teachers-toolkit-index (accessed 6 April 2022).

Reece, I. and Walker, S. (2000). *A Practical Guide to Teaching, Training and Learning*. 4th ed. Tyne and Wear: Business Education Publishers Ltd.

Tiberius, R. (1999). *Small Group Teaching: A Problem Shooting Guide*. London: Kogan Page.

Case-Based Learning

Dr Seri Abraham, Professor Subodh Dave, and Dr Mike Akroyd

Traditionally, medical schools have relied on lecture-based teaching to drive medical education, prior to medical students transitioning into their clinical placements. Over the last two decades, medical schools have been introducing learners to the clinical environment earlier in their medical education. This amalgamation of basic and clinical sciences is known as 'vertical integration'.

Case-based learning (CBL) has been used to bridge the gap between basic science and clinical science as it facilitates integration of a variety of knowledge streams into case vignettes. CBL is a well-established learning approach and has been applied in a variety of professional courses including medicine, dentistry, law and business studies. Within medical education, CBL is used at both undergraduate and postgraduate levels.

Background

It is interesting to note that the approach involving cases to drive learning dates back to the early twentieth century. Professor James Lorrain Smith, Professor in Pathology, introduced the 'case method of teaching pathology' at the University of Edinburgh. He encouraged his students to look up past medical history and cause of death of the deceased patients to corroborate it with the findings of their autopsy (Thistlethwaite, 2015). Over the years, CBL has evolved with the accumulation of experience and evidence in medical education.

CBL is described as an inquiry-based learning method which links theory to practice through the application of knowledge to authentic clinical cases (McLean, 2016).

CBL employs cases to stimulate learning and promotes attainment of knowledge, clinical and non-clinical skills, and attitudes. Cases are produced with a patient background or a clinical situation which is closely aligned to real-life scenarios. In psychiatric cases, supporting information such as past history, risks, collateral information, mental state examination, and investigations may be provided to promote authentic learning. CBL promotes hypothesis generation, team-based collaborative approaches, and integration of learning from other sources – features that it shares with problem-based learning (PBL).

CBL has been considered to have derived from PBL, which involves use of real-life clinical and non-clinical problems to drive learning. Integrated learning, patient-centred learning, project-based learning, and pathway models are some of the other derivatives of PBL. The key difference between PBL and CBL is that PBL eschews the need for prior knowledge or experience of the subject being taught, which may frustrate both trainers and trainees as expertise resident in the trainer is often not utilised. CBL, on the other hand, requires learners to have a degree of prior knowledge and does not necessarily disavow trainers using their clinical expertise in training.

The CBL Process

The process of CBL learning is best understood using the Maastricht 'seven jump' or 'seven step' model. CBL can be undertaken on an individual basis or in a group, either in a classroom or virtually.

Williams' (2005) literature review on applicability of CBL in prehospital education highlights the key steps in CBL:

1. **Clarifying terms:** The case is presented to the learners along with clarification of any terms and concepts which might be new.

2. **Analysis of the case:** Learners use their prior knowledge to recognise problems within the case and reach an agreement regarding events which might need further explanation. The case might have elements intentionally juxtaposed to test the learners' ability to recognise particular clinical and non-clinical concepts: for example, signs and symptoms of serotonin syndrome without explicitly mentioning the syndrome.

3. **Brainstorming:** Learners discuss their pre-existing knowledge regarding the case. Particular emphasis should be placed on individual learners to not comment on the ideas offered by other learners in a group setting. The aim of this step is to offer ideas to structure the problems present in the case. This is a creative process, and a collaborative task when done in groups in a classroom or in a virtual environment. The tutor might take up an active role in this step, particularly when CBL is undertaken on an individual basis.

4. **Formulating learning objectives:** During this step, other members of the group, and the tutor, are allowed to probe pre-existing knowledge and introduce explanations. The aim of this step is to facilitate learners to reach a consensus regarding their own learning objectives. The tutor should ensure that the learning objectives are specific, achievable, relevant, and comprehensive. A state of cognitive dissonance between existing and required knowledge is key to learning. Questions and dilemmas that arise during this step could be used to set learning objectives as part of self-directed learning.

5. **Self-directed learning:** In this step, learners engage in self-directed learning to acquire in-depth knowledge based on the learning objectives. They are expected to explore relevant sources of knowledge with the aim of resolving questions raised in the previous steps. The minimum time for this step is two days, but it could be longer if required.

6. **Synthesis:** Learners share their newly acquired knowledge from self-directed learning. They discuss whether the information gathered provides an accurate and detailed explanation for the issues presented in the case. This provides an opportunity for the tutor to check the learner's decision-making process and correct any misinformation. In a virtual learning environment, discussion forums would be a helpful platform for formulating learning objectives and synthesis of learning.

7. **Feedback:** This includes feedback from the learners and tutor to improve the learning process. This is useful to identify areas for further improvement and integration into clinical practice.

The Role of the Tutor in CBL

The tutor plays a central role as the facilitator in the learning process. The tutor helps guide and support learner (s) through the different steps and beyond. Prior to setting up the session, the tutor should be acquainted with the case, engage in background reading as required, consider various learning outcomes based on the curriculum, and link the knowledge gained with wider learning needs. The tutor might assign various learner roles, such as leader, time keeper, and scribe, to encourage active participation and to place the ownership for learning on the participants.

CBL in a Virtual Environment

CBL can be delivered in a virtual environment in a variety of ways. This could range from uploading the case onto a basic virtual platform to more sophisticated multimedia software that allows multi-user interaction, for example virtual classrooms. Virtual platforms such as Moodle, Articulate, Xerte, etc., aid incorporation of images, texts, and videos into existing templates. Cases can also be linked with quizzes, games, and other learning activities, such as reflections and formative and summative assessments to facilitate deeper and lifelong learning. 'Virtual patients' can be created from the cases to facilitate learners in mastering their clinical and non-clinical skills in a safe environment. Furthermore, virtual patients may be embedded into a virtual hospital or a community with interlinked and/or branching case studies to simulate real-life clinical practice (Jeimy, 2018).

Benefits of CBL

CBL stimulates learners and develops both intrinsic and extrinsic motivation, thereby promoting individualised learning. It also encourages critical reflection, along with integration of knowledge and skills into clinical practice. As mentioned, CBL aids collaborative learning and helps learners achieve a smoother transition into their clinical roles. Learners utilising a CBL approach have shown positive changes in their attitude towards learning as they were able to engage in more meaningful activities as part of their learning and hence found the process more enjoyable (McLean, 2016). There is also some evidence that the CBL approach leads to an improvement in clinical reasoning, diagnostic interpretations, and logical thinking.

Limitations with CBL

Learners may require time to become familiar with the CBL approach if they have not had prior exposure to this. The CBL approach might lead to learners feeling uncertain about their learning needs, and the contextually driven learning style could possibly lead to learners understanding concepts in an erroneous manner. Active input from the tutor would help to manage this. Learners might struggle to relate case-based learning to the theoretical aspect of the subject matter as they might view practical aspects of the cases as separate to theoretical aspects. The interpretive complexities might lead to endless speculation within the learner or group. Particularly pertinent to psychiatry, this might lead to subtle issues – for example, social and cultural aspects of the case being missed and deeper, more complex concepts bypassed or covered in a 'tick box' fashion leading to superficial learning. Guidance from an experienced tutor, relevant self-directed learning, and linking CBL to wider aspects of learning and assessment such as reflections may help overcome these limitations.

Practical Considerations for CBL

1. Developing the content:

   Thistlethwaite (2015) recommends that the cases should follow a storytelling format, with authentic themes closely related to real-life scenarios. The case should be closely aligned to well-defined learning outcomes, have educational value, and stimulate interest. Learners should be able to create empathy with the characters. This could be promoted by telling the story in the present tense, using the patient's voice and direct quotations to add to the realism. The cases should promote decision making and have wide applicability.

   When using CBL, it is important that case libraries reflect the likely real-world presentations. It is the authors' experience that psychiatry elements are often added to other systemic presentations: for example, depression in a patient presenting with gait problems (Parkinson's disease and other movement disorders) rather than reflecting the reality that patients with both physical and mental health problems often present with psychiatric symptoms.

2. **Management of Content**:

   This depends on the platform used to manage and deliver the content. Face-to-face teaching has been managed and delivered via the traditional classroom approach. Virtual platforms could be used for designing, storing, indexing, and referencing the content. This also allows interlinking between cases, learning resources, and external resources using hyperlinks, etc.

3. **Content delivery**:

   This can be undertaken via synchronous delivery, asynchronous delivery, or using a hybrid of both. In synchronous learning, CBL is undertaken in real-time, whereby learner (s) receive and go through the case with the tutor, akin to being in a classroom. This facilitates incorporation of live presentations, webinars, or live simulations into the session. Asynchronous delivery involves the learner (s) accessing the case in their own time and space. Engagement with peers and the tutor is often undertaken directly or virtually using online discussion forums, emails, mobile applications, etc. The advantage with this approach is that learners can access the content in their own time. However, the

---

Box 4.3.1 Key Points When Writing up a Case Study

Your case study should:

Be closely aligned to the curriculum and learning objectives

Follow a story telling format in a structured manner

Arouse the interest of the learner, using dilemmas, conundrums, and issues, provoking conflicting, and facilitating decision making

Include the presence of discrete and possibly branching clinical decision points

Allow learners to analyse the problem-solving options and select a course of action

Encourage assessment and reflection of key learning points

Be easy to link CBL with assessments

(Howlett, 2009)

Box 4.3.2 Take-Home Messages

CBL involves application of theoretical knowledge to clinical practice using clinical cases. This makes it a particularly useful approach for learners transitioning into clinical practice or getting acquainted with a new area of clinical practice.

CBL can be delivered in a variety of ways: individual or group, classroom or virtual; synchronous, asynchronous, or both. This allows flexible learning and widens the scope of application with the approach.

CBL works best when the case is closely aligned to the curriculum and learning objectives. Its effectiveness is further increased by linking the case with structured reflections and assessments to aid lifelong learning.

---

learners need to be motivated to engage and might require additional input from the tutor as compared to a synchronous approach.

4. **Measuring outcomes with CBL:**

The CBL approach has been linked with high student satisfaction levels (Bowe et al., 2009). Furthermore, CBL provides the framework for critical thinking, which helps diagnostic reasoning and clinical decision making (Fortun et al., 2016). Integrative essays, structured reflections, and MCQs were noted to be optimal tools for assessing CBL.

References

Bowe, C. M., Voss, J., and Thomas, A. H. (2009). Case method teaching: An effective approach to integrate the basic and clinical sciences in the preclinical medical curriculum. *Med Teach.* **31** (9): 834–41. https://doi.org/10.1080/01421590902922904

Fortun, J., Morales, A., and Tempest, G. (2017). Introduction and evaluation of case-based learning in the first foundational course of an undergraduate medical curriculum. *Journal of Biological Education*, **51** (3): 295–304.

Howlett, D., Vincent, T., Gainsborough, N., et al. (2009). Integration of a case-based online module into an undergraduate curriculum: What is involved and is it effective? *E-Learning And Digital Media*, **6** (4): 372–84.

Jeimy, S., Wang, J., and Richardson, L. (2018). Evaluation of virtual patient cases for teaching diagnostic and management skills in internal medicine: a mixed methods study. *BMC Research Notes*, **11** (1): 357.

McLean, S. (2016). Case-based learning and its application in medical and health-care fields: A review of worldwide literature. *Journal of Medical Education and Curriculum Development* (vol **3**). https://doi.org/10.4137/JMECD.S20377.

Thistlethwaite, J. (2015). Learning and teaching anatomy through case-based learning (CBL). In L. K. Chan and W. Pawlina (eds.), *Teaching Anatomy* (pp. 125–32). Cham: Springer.

Williams, B. (2005). Case based learning – a review of the literature: Is there scope for this educational paradigm in prehospital education? *Emergency Medicine Journal* **22**: 577–81.

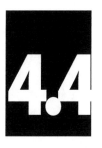

Role Play and Experiential Learning

4.4

Professor Subodh Dave, Dr Seri Abraham, and Dr Mike Akroyd

Kolb's (1984) learning cycle has had a significant influence in shaping medical and psychiatric education. Based on constructivist principles, Kolb emphasises the importance of experiential learning complemented by reflection, abstract conceptualisation, and active experimentation (followed by a repeat of the cycle) as a method of teaching and learning. The influence of experiential learning can be seen in a range of innovations, such as the vertical and horizontal integration of psychiatry in the curriculum, problem-based learning, simulation, role play, vicarious experiencing through films and the arts, and early introduction to clinical experience, to name a few.

Arguably, experiential learning has a more apposite role to play in psychiatric education. Eliciting a patient's real clinical experience relies on the ability of the clinician to find a window into their inner world – hence the importance of *empathy*. This phenomenological approach enables an external assessor to personally experience and access the subjective inner world of the assessee.

Multiple techniques are available to educators to provide this glimpse into the inner world of the patient, namely role play, observed simulations, films, or direct interaction with patients with lived experience of mental illness.

Role Play

Kiger (2004) defined role play as an experiential learning technique using case scenarios involving learners acting out roles to provide practice and gain feedback to improve their skills. It involves use of scenarios based on real-life situations and allows learners to experience both the clinician's and the patient's perspective. While the use of simulated patients (SPs) is effective, ethical, and easy to organise, teaching using SPs can be expensive and less flexible for routine use. Role plays offer a more convenient and accessible form of experiential learning.

Learners take on roles that they are often unfamiliar with and extemporise professional and interpersonal behaviours. Role play is considered to be an invaluable tool for teaching skills, knowledge, and attitudes in clinical and medical education settings. It is also widely used for development of clinical, diagnostic, and interpersonal skills.

Background

The concept of role play in psychiatry was introduced in the 1970s by Scheffler as a method for teaching psychiatric interviewing (Scheffler, 1977). This approach led to reduction in learners' anxiety, better understanding of concepts and skills, and improved identification with patients.

Role play is based on the humanistic and person-centred philosophy of Carl Rogers as it facilitates the learner's ability to understand and experience the feelings and emotions of a patient undergoing mental health difficulties, leading to empathy, reflection, and introspection.

Challenges with Role Play

Role plays are commonly undertaken in an impromptu and unstructured manner, particularly in clinical teaching. This hinders active learning and can lead to reduced satisfaction with the process. Engaging in role play might lead to the feeling of having to perform or of being watched, which can be uncomfortable. Additionally, role play scenarios might trigger emotional memories – for example: traumatic experiences, previous abuse, losses, losing patients to suicide, etc.

Such occurrences would need to be contained sensitively within the session, with follow-up if necessary. Learners might also struggle to get into role-play mode in order to replicate a real-life scenario. This might limit active participation and learning from the session. Debriefing and reflection after the session are key in helping learners analyse the situation and their response, and for consideration of any future modifications they may wish to adopt in dealing with similar situations in future.

Benefits of Role Play in Psychiatric Education

Rønning and Bjørkly (2019) reviewed psychiatric training programmes that had used role play and reflection in psychiatric education and found them to be effective in imparting clinical skills, including communication skills, conducting psychiatric interviews, and eliciting symptoms such as hallucinations. Students learning through role plays not only reported better learning (improved knowledge) but were also more prepared to help people presenting with suicide risk and felt more confident, respectful, and safer in communicating with people presenting with psychiatric problems (improved skills and attitudes).

Role play provides learners with the opportunity to learn, practice, and improve their skills in a safe learning environment, helps evoke interest, and facilitates consolidation of information previously learnt (DeNeve and Heppner, 1997). Furthermore, role play aids transition from the classroom to working in a clinical environment. Engaging in role play provides an immersive experience; allows learners to place themselves in novel situations; and, crucially, helps develop empathy for both patients presenting with psychiatric problems and the clinicians treating them. This helps with the process of self-discovery as learners receive almost instant feedback, and this can be linked up with future learning and reflections. Observing role plays can be a useful learning exercise as well providing a degree of vicarious experience.

Role Play in Virtual Environments

Recently, there has been an exponential increase in virtual learning and this trend is likely to continue in the future. Role play can be undertaken in virtual environments with relative ease. Virtual role play can offer some advantages over face-to-face role plays. In common with other virtual training formats, the cost of running virtual role play sessions is usually lower; moreover, with the advent of technological innovations such as gaming and virtual reality, role play in simulated and virtual worlds is possible, offering the opportunity for immersive and interactive learning experiences. While interaction with bots allows the possibility of virtual role plays, more traditional 'scripted' roles can be conducted with facilitators using email or web-based asynchronous exchanges. It is important to retain fidelity as loss of 'reality' leads to reduced efficacy. Virtual platforms offer relative anonymity and may suit learners who, for a range of reasons, find face-to-face role plays uncomfortable.

The interaction between learners and facilitators is key to learning from role play. Therefore, potential barriers to interaction in a virtual environment should be identified and mitigated prior to delivery. It can be challenging to capture non-verbal communication such as gestures, body language, etc., during virtual role play. It might be useful to acknowledge this limitation at the outset and discuss this as part of the debrief.

Practical Considerations with Setting Up and Running Role Play Sessions

1. Setting up a role play session

   Role play usually has three types of participants: players, facilitators, and observers. A role session can be broken down into three phases: briefing, play, and debriefing.

   The briefing phase usually involves setting out the ground rules and introducing the topic being discussed and the roles. Participants can volunteer for the available roles and seek clarification from the facilitator, as needed. Enough time should be allocated for this. Random allocation using random number generators can address some of the awkwardness associated with volunteering for role plays. Equally, pre-allocating role plays with plenty of notice provides students the opportunity to prepare for the role and also provides plenty of time and opportunity to clarify any issues with the role. Facilitators or course organisers must ensure that students are comfortable with their role. It is also worth bearing in mind that, given the risks of triggering emotions (see earlier discussion), certain students may have a valid reason to be exempt from public role plays. In such cases, educators will need to determine appropriate alternative strategies – for example, a one-to-one observed encounter with a simulated patient.

   The facilitator (s) should ensure that the participants have enough information, resources, and props as needed. Attention must be paid to the seating arrangement for the role players and the observers.

   As the players play their respective roles in the second phase, the facilitator directs the passage of play. The facilitator (s) might choose to take a step back and observe the proceedings and interject, comment, or encourage participation from the role players before withdrawing, as needed. It is helpful to agree in advance whether and how the facilitator (s) will interject. Indeed, for certain learning outcomes, planned pauses with agreed variations in role to enable the experience of variations in outcomes may be helpful.

   The debriefing phase is crucial. The role players talk about their experience of the session and receive feedback from the facilitator (s), other role players, and observers. The facilitator (s) helps the learners identify aspects that went well and areas that need further development. Once again, it is important that it is agreed in advance whether the role players will provide feedback 'in role' or as themselves.

2. Preparation

Adequate preparation is key to running a successful role play session. It would be useful for the facilitator to review feedback from the previous session and ensure that the content of the session is linked to learning objectives, particularly if the scenarios are being reused. Allocating adequate time for each of the three phases, ensuring adherence to time, and regular breaks will promote success with role plays.

As the role play progresses, it takes on a life of its own as it is a dynamic process. Therefore, while preparing for all possible discussion streams is advisable, particularly for the initial scenarios in the sessions, it is also vital to prepare participants for unanticipated departures from the script. The facilitator should be sensitive to the emotional content of the scenarios and to the impact of the learner's social, cultural, or religious background. In all cases, the facilitator must have clear, predefined indicators to signal an immediate pause to the role play. Debriefing is particularly vital in such scenarios.

3. Creating role play scenarios

Role plays need to be designed carefully, keeping in mind the twin objectives of ensuring fidelity to both real life and to desired learning outcomes. A useful strategy for educators is to draw up a bank of case scenarios targeting key learning outcomes, which may be based around specific mental health conditions (e.g. depression, anxiety, dementia, etc.) or based on presentations (distress, agitation, confusion, risky behaviour, etc.). These core scenarios can then be altered and tailored to different learning outcomes: for example, the age of the patient, the location of the patient (GP surgery, outpatient clinic, emergency department, etc.), additional physical and/or mental comorbidity, etc. Additional layers of complexity incur incorporating themes pertaining to legal conundrums, cultural aspects, and ethical and professional dilemmas to ensure that they deliver learners' needs. Well-structured role plays have the right amount of relevant information to ensure a high level of fidelity without compromising on ease of use.

Highly structured, less complex and low-fidelity scenarios are probably easier to start the session with, but as the learners get to grips with the approach, a transition into less structured, complex, and high-fidelity scenarios will help the learners gain a deeper understanding of and mastery over the subject (Joyner and Young, 2006).

4. Encourage participation and co-production

Learners should be encouraged to actively participate in the session. Varying and switching roles helps engagement and helps students get both the patient and the clinician perspective but also, from an educational viewpoint, helps them get a sense of the examiners' frame of reference. Allowing observers to be examiners and actively involving them in discussion helps with engagement and learning.

Use of open questions and a reflective approach generally aids participation. The facilitator should consider seeking feedback from learners regarding the process and the content of the session to help identify areas that could be improved. Further avenues for co-production should be sought from learners displaying clinical and cultural expertise in clinical and non-clinical areas covered during the session.

5. Linking up with wider learning

Learners are likely to benefit more when role play is linked to wider aspects of learning, based on curriculum requirements. Learners should be asked to identify two to three areas for further self-directed or guided learning. Learning could be consolidated by supplementary reflections, peer discussion, and more role-play-based learning with the aim of smooth transition into clinical spaces.

Role Play: Assessment and Evaluation

Role plays are often used for formative assessment. A structured assessment approach is often used for providing feedback for participants and observers. It is useful to incorporate key features of both process and content in the tool. Moreover, such tools can also be used as an active observation tool enabling observers to rate their peers and learn at the same time.

Generic Likert scale-based tools with free-text boxes for comments can be helpful in obtaining pertinent feedback from students. Course organisers should build routine analysis of this feedback into their course evaluation strategy to enable tweaks to the role play or assessment tools if needed.

Box 4.4.1 Take-Home Points

Role play is a valuable experiential learning tool for improving clinical and non-clinical skills in a safe environment.

Fidelity to real-life scenarios, incorporating themes with increasing complexity, followed by facilitated reflection leads to effective learning through role play.

References

DeNeve, K. M. and Heppner, M. J. (1977). Role play simulations: The assessment of an active learning technique and comparisons with traditional lectures. *Innov High Educ.*, **21**: 231–46.

Joyner, B. and Young, L. (2006). Teaching medical students using role play: Twelve tips for successful role plays. *Medical Teacher*, **28** (3): 225–9.

Kiger, A. (2004). *Teaching for Health*. 3rd ed. Edinburgh: Churchill Livingstone.

Kolb, D. A. (1984). *Experiential learning: Experience as the source of learning and development.* Englewood Cliffs, NJ: Prentice Hall.

Rønning, S. B. and Bjørkly, S. (2019). The use of clinical role-play and reflection in learning therapeutic communication skills in mental health education: An integrative review. *Adv Med Educ Pract.* **10**: 415–25.

Scheffler, L. W. (1977). Being is believing: Playing the psychiatric patient. *J Psychiatr Educ.* **1** (1): 63–7.

Simulation

Dr Mike Akroyd, Professor Subodh Dave, and Dr Seri Abraham

What is Simulation?

Simulation has been described as 'the artificial replication of sufficient components of a real-world situation to achieve certain goals' (Gaba, qtd in Ziv, Small, and Wolpe, 2000, p. 57). Simulation goes back hundreds of years, with references to mock battles and rehearsal of hunting rituals. In the modern era, the aviation industry, the military, and others professions associated with risk have used simulation for decades in order to help individuals and teams to build confidence and competence (Rosen, 2008).

Applying simulation to healthcare is not a recent phenomenon. In France and Italy in the eighteenth century, du Coudray and Galli respectively introduced birthing simulators in order to teach techniques associated with childbirth (RMK Aimes, 2017). During the twentieth century, rapid technological developments gave simulation a role in increasingly more complicated situations, typified by the launch of Resusci-Anne in the 1960s, which, following the introduction of a spring into the chest, went on to be the most commonly used manikin for teaching of cardiopulmonary resuscitation worldwide. This was closely followed by 'Harvey', the cardiology patient simulator, which could vary pulse, blood pressure, heart sounds, etc., in order to depict a large number of cardiac disorders. Manikins have continued to develop in tandem with other advances in healthcare, and today can be intubated, cannulated, catheterised, and even allow intraosseous insertions.

This is not to say that all simulation relies on technology. In 1964, Howard Barrows started to use actors in order to depict clinical presentations, simulating signs and symptoms of a range of disorders (Barrows, 1968). This concept of the 'simulated patient' – a person without any real clinical signs or symptoms trained to portray a particular role to facilitate teaching or assessment (Ker, 2007) – was extended to the 'standardised patient': a simulated/actual patient trained to portray their symptoms in a consistently replicable way for teaching and assessment by the Canadian psychometrician Geoffrey Norman (Collins, 1998). In the 1970s, actors began to be used to construct challenging situations, such as a patient who presents as overtly hostile, reticent, or seductive. In 1975, Harden introduced simulated patients played by actors into objective structured clinical examinations (OSCEs), and their use in undergraduate and postgraduate medical education is now commonplace (Eagles et al., 2007).

In mental health, as with all aspects of healthcare, there is a huge amount of learning that takes place in the course of provision of care. Kolb's educational theory based on the constructive cycle of experience and reflection, followed by analysis and experimentation, fits well with the traditional models of medical education of apprenticeship or preceptorship, a process that starts with didactic learning, progressing to observation and then performance under supervision. This is in keeping with Osler's view that medicine was 'learned by the bedside and not in the classroom' (Kolb, 1984; Peters and Ten Cate, 2014). Medical education has been described as a form of socialisation or 'professional identity development' (Jarvis-Selinger et al., 2012, p. 1185), with gradual transition into the clinical environment.

However, in the real world such concrete experiences appear opportunistically, and active experimentation can only go so far in settings where the needs of the patient necessarily take priority. In the simulation setting, learning experiences can be controlled and standardised. In stark contrast to real-life situations, the needs of the learner can be paramount. Participants can try (and sometimes retry) different approaches, and the impact of clinical decisions taken in this setting can 'played out', safe in the knowledge that there are no real-life patients being exposed to potential risk.

There is a growing evidence-base in support of the use of simulation in the teaching of procedural skills, teamwork, and communication, and it is seen as an important way to address the disconnect 'between the classroom and the clinical environment' (Okuda et al., 2009, p. 330). It is promoted as an effective learning tool by Health Education England (2019), the Department of Health (2011), the General Medical Council (2015), and the Nursing and Midwifery Council (2019). Reviews of untoward incidents in healthcare frequently identify communication, decision making, situational awareness, and other 'human factors' as problematic (Reason, 1995), and simulation training can provide a means of exploring and addressing such issues. The publication 'Safer Medical Practice' (Department of Health, 2008) referred to high-profile situations in the aviation industry wherein use of simulation had been of significant benefit, and went on to identify areas where it could have prevented adverse outcomes in healthcare.

Why Use Simulation in Psychiatry?

There has been a historical perception within mental health that simulation was in some way more suited to specialties where technical procedures are common, and hence 'not (for) us' (Jordan, 2012, p. 26). A 2008 literature review of simulation in psychiatric education commented that use of this tool had been taken up 'in a somewhat random fashion' (McNaughton et al., 2008, p. 86). Where simulation did exist in psychiatry, much of this had emerged as a way of preparing for the most common use of simulation and role play: the OSCE.

In more recent years, there has been a growing interest in the potential applications of simulation within psychiatry, particularly in situations where there could otherwise be barriers to experiential learning. Simulation is recognised as a way to teach not only psychiatric and other transferable skills, but also desirable behaviours and attitudes (Dave, 2012). Broadly speaking, use of simulation in psychiatry falls into two main groups: the teaching of advanced communication skills and exposure to specific clinical situations.

Advanced Communication Skills

Coyle, Miller, and McGowen (1998) considered the difficulties associated with teaching skills related to psychotherapy, including the inherent lack of predictability in the emergence of learning opportunities and the fact that the nature of interactions in psychotherapy means that supervision can often occur some time after the interaction itself. They developed a number of standardised patient scripts, structured to ensure the emergence of the concepts identified as learning objectives ('identifying feelings, understanding family dynamics, challenging irrational ideas'; p. 591), and enlisted mental health professionals as simulated patients. Two learners would act as co-therapists, whilst other learners observed. Interactions between the learners and the simulated patients were followed by a longer debrief, with feedback from peers, faculty staff, and the simulated patients themselves. Klamen and Yudkowsky (2002) developed this idea further, using standardised patients who were invited to use and build upon their own personal history in order to enhance fidelity. Learners were then invited to conduct an initial psychodynamic psychotherapy session. This taped encounter was used as part of discussions with the wider group in a debrief, something that would not be possible with real-life patient interactions. Clay et al. (2000) used similar ideas in teaching skills relating to family therapy, and others have used simulation to address complex clinical ethics scenarios (Edinger et al., 1999).

Exposure to Specific Clinical Situations

In inpatient mental health settings, complex physical comorbidities, the use of potent psychotropic medication, and the overlay of symptoms of mental disorder can make physical health emergencies more likely to arise. Some of the more serious emergencies are fortunately relatively rare, although this makes it even less likely that junior staff will have direct access to senior supervision the first time that they are confronted with them in real life. In Yorkshire and the Humber (Akroyd, Jordan, and Rowlands, 2016) and at St Thomas's Hospital, London (Thomson et al., 2013), simulation has been used to give doctors or multidisciplinary teams the opportunity to practice the recognition, assessment, and initial management of physical health problems that can occur in psychiatry. Scenarios were written based upon real-life untoward incidents, such as over-sedation following rapid tranquilisation, Wernicke's encephalopathy, and neuroleptic malignant syndrome. Learners, given a small amount of initial information and access to other 'props' such as case notes and prescription records, would interact with their patient (an actor, a high-fidelity manikin, or sometimes a combination of the two) in real time, with a longer debrief afterwards, focussing on non-technical skills and human factors.

What Are the Challenges Associated with Simulation?

Expertise

Learning in a simulated setting places the needs of the learner as the primary concern. Scenarios are standardised in order to make a desired outcome or outcomes emerge, allowing for incorrect or even dangerous outcomes in real life to be 'played out'. Debriefing for the wider group of learners offers the opportunity for true learning, helping them identify and close gaps in knowledge and skills (Raemer et al., 2011). Facilitation of this type takes skill and expertise, and to facilitate without this can seriously impact upon learning. Such an approach must itself be learnt and practised, and is a departure from more familiar and common approaches, such as those involving Pendleton's guidelines (Timmis and Speirs, 2015).

Engagement with the Approach

There are reports of situations where the nature of simulation itself has been felt to be a barrier to engagement of the learners. Krahn et al. (2002) presented trained standardised patients to a group of actual patients involved in a course introducing postgraduates to psychopathology. They found that learners were generally able to identify those who were standardised, and that they felt less empathetic and less attentive towards them. They inferred that a sense of 'being tricked' on the part of the learners could interfere with an ability to engage in an empathetic manner or encourage enacting empathy rather than feeling empathy. Issues such as these can themselves emerge through the debriefing process. Brenner (2009) was of the view that whilst simulation could be useful in teaching specific, discrete skills, its use in teaching related to psychotherapy and more complex interpersonal skills was more problematic.

Cost

Cost has also been identified as a potential barrier to more widespread adoption of simulation in healthcare (Curtis, DiazGranados, and Feldman, 2012). In mental health, where simulation is perhaps less likely to require more advanced technological simulation equipment than some medical specialties, there can nevertheless be significant costs involved in the initial set-up and ongoing running of simulation. In order to provide immersive, true-to-life experiences for learners, simulation can involve the use of high-fidelity manikins and medical actors, and even the development of dedicated simulation suites. In addition to this, the nature of simulation is such that small-group teaching is necessary, with a high ratio of instructors to learners (Datta, Upadhyay, and Jaideep, 2012).

Set-up and Running of Simulation

Construction of Scenarios

Harrington and Simon (2020) consider simulation design as akin to a professional stage production, where the faculty are the writers and directors, education specialists (and sometimes simulation technicians) are the production staff, and the learners are the audience. Extending this analogy, they stress the importance of scenario design templates or 'storyboarding' as tools to help in envisaging how a scenario can play out, considering the intended learning outcomes within the desired context. They highlight the need to provide guidance in five key areas:

1. Guidance for scenario facilitators: This should include a summary of the simulated case, the key learning objectives, and a proposed flow of the scenario, as well as anticipated diversions or learner mistakes.
2. Technical guidance: This needs to cover necessary equipment, including manikins, moulage, any props, and whether actors are required.
3. Roles/scripts: There needs to be guidance for standardised or simulated patients about what to say, how to behave, and how to react to the anticipated actions or words of the learners.
4. Debriefing: There should be emphasis on the learning objectives to be revisited as part of debriefing, and this may be supplemented by guidance on the principles identified in the section on 'Debriefing'.
5. Final planning: Those involved in delivery of simulation should meet to discuss their shared understanding of each of the above components, and consider running the

scenario as a 'dress rehearsal' prior to learners being invited to participate. This is likely to highlight any changes that need to be made.

Debriefing

It has been said that simulation scenarios are essentially 'a good excuse to debrief' (Gardner, 2013, p. 168) and, quite understandably, debrief is described as 'the heart and soul of the simulation experience' (Rall, Manser, and Howard, 2009, p. 516), enabling reflection and genesis of alternative skills that can be practised in high-fidelity simulated situations.

Whilst a range of debriefing approaches exist, they have key components in common. Rudolph et al. (2006) considered three important phases in debriefing: the 'reactions phase', the 'understanding phase', and the 'summary phase'.

The 'reactions phase' is an opportunity for initial emotional reactions to be shared and aired. This is likely to highlight the matters that learners are most concerned about. Whilst there is often a lot of self-criticism on the part of learners, this also provides the opportunity for facilitators to put things into perspective, perhaps sharing that they have acted similarly or seen similar actions taken before by others. Importantly, this reinforces the notion that there is a 'safe space' for the open discussion of decisions and behaviours. Once there is a shared appreciation amongst the group of exactly *what* took place, it is possible to explore *why*.

In this 'understanding phase', facilitators state a perspective, and follow this up with a question, known as an 'advocacy-inquiry' approach. They open with a first-person perception: 'I saw', 'I noticed', 'I was happy'; then they follow this with curiosity: 'what' or 'why'. A facilitator may say 'I noticed that you asked about suicidal ideation after he disclosed ideas of aggression. What was going through your mind at the time?' or 'I heard you say to the patient that you were going to override their confidentiality and raise a safeguarding concern. Why did you say that?' This approach can help to elicit the thoughts, feelings, and experiences of the learners in order to build a more complex understanding of the experience being discussed and emphasise a sense of collaboration in the solving of the problem at hand.

In the 'summary phase', the facilitator helps learners to share their take-home lessons from the experience and consider what sort of things they did well, as well as what they may do differently next time and what they may have to change if the situation occurred within their clinical practice.

Conclusions

Simulation is an established part of medical education. Whilst it has taken longer to become embedded within psychiatry than in other medical specialities, interest in this approach has helped it to grow, particularly when it comes to helping to address learning objectives around advanced communication skills or those related to uncommon or unpredictable clinical situations. There are clear advantages to allowing learners to practice approaches to a range of clinical encounters in a way that eliminates potential risk to patients. However, in order for simulation to be done well, there needs to be sufficient investment in terms of faculty input and development, as well as commitment to cover of associated costs, not least release of staff for small-group learning.

Box 4.5.1 Key Messages

- Simulation is about giving learners the opportunity to participate in a clinical encounter, acting as they normally would in their clinical practice.
- These encounters can take any form, ranging from the common (e.g. an initial psychotherapy assessment) to rarer situations (e.g. identification of neuroleptic malignant syndrome), where there are inherent barriers to supported experiential learning.
- In stark contrast to clinical practice, the needs of the learner are allowed to be paramount. This gives learners the licence to make mistakes, without exposing patients to avoidable harm.
- Simulated scenarios must be followed by a facilitated debrief, to talk through the emergent learning.
- Debriefing with good judgement, using an advocacy-inquiry approach, allows the perspectives of participants, observers, and facilitators to be discussed openly, leading to deeper understanding of what led to decisions being made, and as such provides greater opportunity for exploration of other approaches.

References

Akroyd, M., Jordan, G., and Rowlands, P. (2016). Interprofessional, simulation-based technology-enhanced learning to improve physical healthcare in psychiatry: The RAMPPS course. *Health Informatics Journal*, 22 (2): 397–405.

Alty, A. (2008). Nurses' learning experience and expressed opinions regarding seclusion practice within one NHS trust. *Journal of Advanced Nursing*, 25 (4): 786–93.

Barrows, H. S. (1968). Simulated patients in medical teaching. *Canadian Medical Association Journal*, 98, 674–6.

Brenner, A. M. (2009). Uses and limitations of simulated patients in psychiatric education. *Academic Psychiatry*, 33, 112–19.

Clay, M. C., Lane, H., Willis, S. E., Peal, M., Chakravarthi, S., and Poehlman, G. (2000). Using a standardized family to teach clinical skills to medical students. *Teaching and Learning in Medicine*, 12 (3): 145–9.

Collins, J. and Harden, R. (1998). AMEE Medical Education Guide No. 13: Real patients, simulated patients and simulators in clinical examinations. *Medical Teacher* 20: 508–21.

Coyle, B., Miller, M., and McGowen, K. R. (1998). Using standardized patients to teach and learn psychotherapy. *Academic Medicine*, 73 (5): 591–2.

Curtis, M. T., DiazGranados, D., and Feldman, M. (2012). Judicious use of simulation technology in continuing medical education. *Journal of Continuing Education in the Health Professions*, **32** (4): 255–60.

Datta, R., Upadhyay, K. K., and Jaideep, C. N. (2012). Simulation and its role in medical education. *Medical Journal, Armed Forces India*, **68** (2): 167–72.

Dave, S. (2012). Simulation in psychiatric teaching. *Advances in Psychiatric Treatment*, **18** (4): 292–8.

Department of Health. (2008). *CMO annual report 2008 – Safer medical practice: Machines, manikins and polo mints*. London: Department of Health.

Department of Health. (2011). *A framework for technology enhanced learning: Report no. 16787*. London: Department of Health.

Department of Health. (2015). *Mental Health Act 1983: Code of Practice*. Norwich: The Stationery Office.

Eagles, J. M., Calder, S. A., Wilson, S., Murdoch, J. M., and Sclare, P. D. (2007). Simulated patients in undergraduate education in psychiatry. *Psychiatric Bulletin*, **31**, 187–90.

Edinger, W., Robertson, J., Skeel, J., and Schoonmaker, J. (1999). Using standardized patients to teach clinical ethics. *Medical Education Online*, **4** (1): 1–5.

Gardner, R. (2013). Introduction to debriefing. *Seminars in Perinatology*, **37** (3): 166–74.

General Medical Council. (2015). Promoting Excellence: Standards for Medical Education and Training. Available at: General Medical Council: www.gmc-uk.org/-/media/documents/promoting-excellence-standards-for-medical-education-and-training-2109_pdf-61939165.pdf (accessed 27 March 2022).

Harrington, D. W. and Simon, L. V. (2020). Designing a Simulation Scenario. Available at: StatPearls: www.ncbi.nlm.nih.gov/books/NBK547670/.

Health Education England. (2019). Simulation. Available at: Health Education England: www.hee.nhs.uk/our-work/simulation.

Jarvis-Selinger, S., Pratt, D. D., and Regehr, G. (2012). Competency is not enough: Integrating identity formation into the medical education discourse. *Academic Medicine*, **87** (9): 1185–90.

Jordan, G. (2012). *Mental health and learning disabilities: The physical health agenda achieved through training, education and simulation.* Leeds: Health Education Yorkshire and the Humber.

Ker, J. and Bradley, P. (2007). *Simulation in Medical Education: Understanding Medical Education.* Association for the Study of Medical Education.

Klamen, D. L. and Yudkowsky, R. (2002). Using standardized patients for formative feedback in an Introduction to Psychotherapy course. *Academic Psychiatry*, **26**, 168–72.

Kolb, D. A. (1984). *Experiential learning: Experience as the source of learning and development.* Englewood Cliffs, NJ: Prentice Hall.

Krahn, L. E., Bostwick, J. M., Sutor, B., and Olsen, M. W. (2002). The challenge of empathy: A pilot study of the use of standardized patients to teach introductory psychopathology to medical students. *Academic Psychiatry*, **26**, 26–30.

Kunkler, K. (2006). The role of medical simulation: An overview. *The International Journal of Medical Robotics and Computer Assisted Surgery* **2**, 203–210.

McNaughton, N., Ravitz, P., Wadell, A., and Hodges, B. D. (2008). Psychiatric education and simulation: A review of the literature. *Canadian Journal of Psychiatry*, **53** (2): 85–93.

Nursing and Midwifery Council. (2019). Different Learning Opportunities. Available at: Nursing and Midwifery Council: www.nmc.org.uk/supporting-information-on-standards-for-student-supervision-and-assessment/learning-environments-and-experiences/types-of-learning-experiences/different-learning-opportunities/

Okuda, Y., Bryson, E. O., DeMaria Jr, S., et al. (2009). The utility of simulation in medical education: What is the evidence. *Mount Sinai Journal of Medicine*, **76** (4): 330–43.

Peters, M. and Ten Cate, O. (2014). Bedside teaching in medical education: A literature review. *Perspectives on Medical Education*, **3** (2): 76–8.

Phrampus, P. (2016). Learning from Simulation – Far more than the Debriefing. Available at: Simulating Healthcare: https://simulatinghealthcare.net/2016/04/25/learning-from-simulation-far-more-than-the-debriefing/.

Raemer, D., Anderson, M., Cheng, A., Fanning, R., Nadkami, V., and Savoldelli, G. (2011). Research regarding debriefing as part of the learning process. *Simulation in Healthcare*, **6**, S52–7.

Rall, M., Manser, T., and Howard, S. K. (2009). Key elements of debriefing for simulator training. *European Journal of Anaesthesiology*, **17** (8): 516–17.

Reason, J. (1995). Understanding adverse events: Human factors. *Quality Health Care*, **4** (2): 80–9.

RMK Aimes. (2017). *About RMK Aimes.* Available at: www.aimes.org/en/page/about-us/history-of-simulation

Rosen, K. (2008). The history of medical simulation. *Journal of Critical Care*, **23** (2): 157–66.

Rudolph, J. W., Simon, R., Dufresne, R. L., and Raemer, D. B. (2006). There's no such thing as 'nonjudgmental' debriefing: A theory and method for debriefing with good judgment. *Simulation in Healthcare*, **1** (1): 49–55.

Thomson, A. B., Cross, S., Key, S., Jaye, P., and Iversen, A. C. (2013). How we developed an emergency psychiatry training course for new residents using principles of high-fidelity simulation. *Medical Teacher*, **35** (10): 797–800.

Timmis, C. and Speirs, K. (2015). Student perspectives on post-simulation debriefing. *The Clinical Teacher*, **12** (6): 418–22.

Ziv, A., Small, S. D., and Wolpe, P. R. (2000). Patient safety and simulation-based medical education. *Medical Teacher*, **22** (5): 489–95.

4.6

Balint Groups for Medical Students

Dr Angeliki Zoumpouli and Dr Barbara Wood

Introduction

There has been increasing emphasis on reflective practice throughout the NHS and in medical training, and this is cited as an essential skill by the General Medical Council (GMC). There are many different models of reflective practice but that one currently being used for medical students across the United Kingdom is the Balint model. Balint groups employ a particular structured approach to reflective practice and focus on the emotional aspects of the doctor–patient or student–patient relationship. The structure of the groups and the stance of the leadership create a space to think about patients holistically, to explore how the patient may be feeling and the feelings that the patient evokes in the presenter and the group members, and increases their understanding of patients' communications.

In 2014, the Royal College of Psychiatrists set up a working group to promote the development of medical student psychotherapy and Balint group schemes across the country. Around 50% of all medical schools in the United Kingdom now offer Balint groups to students, most in their first year of clinical training. King's College London GKT (Guy's, King's and St Thomas') School of Medical Education is the largest medical school in Europe and our experience has developed from running Balint groups for more than 600 third-year students between 2017 and 2020.

The Balint Model of Reflective Practice

Balint groups were developed by the medical doctor and psychoanalyst Michael Balint and his wife Enid in the 1950s and were first described in the book *The Doctor, his Patient and the Illness* (1957). Such groups consist of around ten participants and one or two leaders; they follow a particular structure and run for between 50–60 minutes for medical student groups. The group starts with a reminder about confidentiality and an invitation for someone to present an encounter with a patient that has made an impact on them and stayed in their mind. The presentation, lasting up to 10 minutes, includes a description of the encounter, feelings evoked, and some background history. The presentation is informal, not necessitating any notes or a specific structure, unlike presentations in most other medical settings. The group is invited to ask factual, clarifying questions for a few minutes and then the presenter sits back and listens to the discussion, rejoining 10–15 minutes before the end of the session. The discussion is 'free floating' and focuses on the relationship between the doctor or student and the patient, paying particular attention to emotional aspects. Relationships between the patient, their 'illness', the wider treating team, and family dynamics may also be considered.

Balint groups follow certain 'rules', the overall purpose of which is to provide a safe and confidential space, helping the group to feel more secure and thus allowing more freedom to

Table 4.6.1 Rules of Balint groups

Ground rules	Balint rules
Confidentiality	Excluding latecomers who have missed much of the presentation
Respect	Use of term 'presenter'
Time keeping Starting and finishing on time	Presenting without notes
Notification of absences	Questions of clarification (limited to around 5 minutes)
Refraining from using mobiles/ laptops/tablets (face-to-face groups)	Presenter sitting back after presenting and answering clarifying questions

think, play with ideas, and learn. There are general ground rules which are common to and implicit in most professional group endeavours, and rules more specific to Balint group work (Table 4.6.1). Rules will inevitably be bent or broken, but attention and thought to how and why this happens can be helpful. For example, is this being done reasonably and mindfully under the circumstances, or are facilitators bowing to pressure to avoid the work of the group.

Starting on time and excluding latecomers is not intended punitively, but latecomers may distract the group, will miss the presentation, and will not be in a place to join in the discussion. This also emphasises that everyone's presence and view is important and all have a responsibility to attend.

Use of the term 'presenter' rather than the student's name reminds the group that this is about their professional development *not* the personal characteristics of the student presenting. It reduces the risk of moving into 'therapy' for the presenter and so disrupting the focus of the group. It also provides some protection to the presenter, who may easily expose themselves more than they might wish.

The informal presentation without notes allows for a freer, more fluid and 'alive' portrayal of the interaction and for the subsequent discussion. It produces a different atmosphere in a group discussion where not knowing something is not reprehensible but a matter for exploration. There can be unexpected emphases and surprising omissions in the presentation which may be significant to the case.

Questions of clarification are about matters of fact not of process. They are best limited to around 5 minutes as otherwise the group can continue to interrogate the presenter rather than work on the material given. The most important issues are often revealed early in the presentation, and more questions and information can obscure rather than enlighten.

The aim of the presenter sitting back is to protect them from continued questioning by the group and to help the group focus on the information already given. It also offers the presenter an opportunity to think about their case in the light of the discussion.

Themes in Medical Student Balint Groups

The themes that typically come up in medical student Balint groups include feelings evoked by patients (Torppa et al., 2008), attitudes of and towards doctors, managing and treating patients, and the role of the medical student (Table 4.6.2).

Table 4.6.2 Themes that typically emerge in medical student Balint groups

Feelings evoked by patients	Attitudes of and towards doctors	Managing and treating patients	Medical student role
Sense that medical professionals should always have positive feelings towards patients and difficulty in acknowledging more complex or negative feelings	Disappointment about the absence of a holistic view and of consideration of psychosocial factors of illness	Coping with failures and the limits of medical treatment	Is the role that of a friend, a confidant, or a doctor? How to establish professional boundaries with a patient?
When difficult feelings arise how these can be used to help understand the patient?	Doctors being experienced as cold and unempathetic towards patients (including not listening and withholding information)	Dealing with uncertainty	Developing a sense of professional identity: what kind of doctor do they want to become?
Patients can remind one of oneself, one's own family, or friends; what are the implications of this?	Beliefs that doctors can find situations distressing and perform better if they are less attuned to their patient and their interactions with them	What is it like for the patient's family and friends?	Appreciating help from patients, guilt at 'using' patients for one's own learning
To what extent are difficult feelings also related to doctors or medical students' personal lives and internal worlds?		Considering psychosomatic aspect of illness	Fear of contact with mental health patients, will you make them worse? Fear of risk of suicide
		Breaking bad news	

Leadership of Balint Groups for Medical Students

There are important differences between running Balint groups for experienced clinicians compared with groups for medical students who will not have had experience of this type of work previously. Modifications in technique include greater encouragement and more involvement in the discussion whilst also being mindful of the leadership role and of providing space for the group to develop. Whilst the focus is on patient encounters, students bring broader concerns of emotional relevance, for example of their development as future doctors, which should be accommodated.

Other challenges in leading groups for students relate to their youth, their limited exposure to clinical work, and that participation in a Balint group is usually a novel and very different learning experience for them, which can feel threatening given their greater familiarity with didactic, science-focussed teaching. Leaders need to be sensitive to where the students are developmentally and the related difficulties they may face in this work. Students are often very anxious to start with and some may easily feel humiliated. They may have concerns about being scrutinised psychologically, especially by psychiatrist facilitators, and there may be an idea that this is some kind of group therapy. Some students will be less receptive to this experience and need more encouragement, especially when the groups are a mandatory requirement of their training.

Balint groups are usually located in psychiatry placements and led by trainee and/or consultant psychiatrists, which can lead to them being viewed as less relevant to the rest of medical practice. It is important to counter this view by making it clear that presentations of non-psychiatric cases are welcomed (Table 4.6.3).

Co-leadership

Having two co-leaders has some advantages. This can be a helpful way to model and offer the group a 'reflective pair' and can provide the group with greater containment. It also can provide diversity as there are likely to be differences in professional interests and/or gender, racial, and cultural identity. The perceived or actual seniority relationships in the co-leadership pair can benefit the group through respectful and creative ways of relating to one another and by offering students different role models with whom to identify. A co-leadership pair can model a difference in opinion or approach which engenders curiosity rather than conflict. Co-leadership also allows sharing of the leaders' responsibilities: for example, keeping to the structure and timings, attending to the emotional tone of the group, and helping students maintain focus on emotional and relational aspects.

However, co-leadership is not without its challenges. There may be differences in approach and personality that result in difficulties in finding a pace and working harmoniously together. One leader may feel scrutinised by or inferior to their co-leader, which can cause inhibition in the group. Co-leaders can get caught up in their own exchanges, which can be unhelpful to students if too prolonged. Due to these challenges, supervision is important to provide a space to think about the Balint group and the dynamics between group members and the leaders but also between the co-leaders.

The Benefits of Balint Groups for Medical Students

Training in medicine is challenging, involving not only major academic and clinical skills components but also increasing exposure to the impact of illness and dying and to

Table 4.6.3 Balint Group Leadership

General Group Management	Work of a Balint Group	Specific Problems and Techniques
Keep to time	Help the group to keep its primary focus on the student (doctor/team)–patient relationship	Help the group from moving towards other clinical and management issues - 'what is going on?' not 'what to do?'
Remind about confidentiality	Remind the group the purpose is for emotional and relational considerations	Intervene to protect group members from unwanted personal questioning
Monitor feelings of the group and its members	Encourage reflection on how the patient may feel and on how the patient makes us feel	Manage excessive personal disclosure
Help the group manage distress	Represent those in danger of being lost – especially the patient	Prioritise facilitating rather than joining the discussion as a member
Make space for quieter people to speak	Allow reflection on feelings and relationships in the patient's family and the wider treating team	Reflect questions
Allow the group to follow preferred lines of thought (within limits)	Allow medical students space to consider other areas of emotional relevance to them	Observe and draw attention to metaphors
Tolerate uncertainty and silence (within limits)		Note parallel process – group discussion reflecting what was happening in the patient encounter

interpersonal encounters with patients which can evoke strong emotions in the student doctor. This all happens in parallel with students having to forge their own professional identity and during young adulthood, which in itself poses significant internal and external developmental challenges.

Participation in a Balint group provides students with an opportunity to talk about and explore the emotional and interpersonal aspects of work with patients. The process of reflection encourages students to develop a more holistic approach to medical practice and develop a better understanding of patients' communication so patients become more interesting to listen to and easier to help.

Students may realise that certain patients or emotions resonate with what is going on in their own inner and outer lives. Although this may be difficult to manage, the students can learn to reflect on this and turn it to therapeutic advantage. Increasing emotional awareness and attention to the psychological pressures of practicing medicine through participation in group reflection can reduce burn out and harmful coping mechanisms and increase resilience and enjoyment of the privilege as well as the challenges of medical practice.

In addition, doctors work in team environments and need to develop interpersonal proficiencies and some awareness of group dynamics in order to do so effectively. Participating in Balint groups helps students develop crucial skills in listening to and respecting the views and feelings of others and in discussing situations where there are no clear-cut answers that are common in all areas of medicine.

Literature Showing that Balint Groups are Effective

There is growing evidence that Balint groups provide a facilitative environment wherein empathy can be built and wherein the complexities of patients as human beings can be embraced. Airagnes et al. (2014) compared 34 medical students who participated in Balint groups with 129 students who did not. Students involved in the Balint groups demonstrated enhanced empathy as measured on the interpersonal reactivity index (IRI). They were also asked to rate their emotional responses to two case-reports with relational difficulties; again, only students in the Balint group showed enhanced empathy, and they were also more able to consider the affective dimension of the doctor–patient relationship (Airagnes et al., 2014).

Following this preliminary study, Du Vaure et al. (2017) conducted a randomised controlled trial where fourth-year medical students were allocated to a Balint group or a control group: 155 students in the intervention group were compared to 144 in the control group, with no differences in baseline measures. The intervention group displayed significantly higher empathy on the Jefferson's School Empathy Scale – Medical Student (JSPE-MS©) at follow-up compared with the control group (p=0.002).

Yazdankhahfard et al. (2019) conducted a systematic review of research publications on Balint groups in medical education between 2008 and 2018. Qualitative studies suggested that Balint groups play an important role in personal and professional development and also help medical students to understand the impact of their own personality on their consultations with patients. The quantitative studies (n=4) indicated that participation in Balint groups increases students' understanding of the doctor–patient relationship and improves their communication skills (Yazdankhahfard et al., 2019). A study of forty third-year medical students participating in Balint groups at King's College London in 2017/18 showed a significant increase in empathy scores (p< 0.05) across the group, with the largest increases in the subgroup of students with lower empathy scores before the Balint group experience (Dr Ben Robinson – personal communication/preparation for publication).

Currently, research is being carried out on medical student cohorts starting their first clinical year in 2020 at a national level in the United Kingdom, looking at the effects of participation in Balint groups on empathy, compassion, resilience, and burnout, and whether participating in Balint groups influences the choice of a future career among the medical specialities.

References

Airagnes, G., Consoli, S. M., De Morlhon, O., Galliot, A-M. Lemogne, C., and Jaury, P. (2014). Appropriate training based on Balint groups can improve the empathic abilities of medical students: A preliminary study *Journal of Psychosomatic Research* **76**: 426–9.

Balint, M. (1957). *The Doctor, His Patient and the Illness*. International Universities Press.

Du Vaure, C. B., Lemogne, C., Bunge, L., et al. (2017). Promoting empathy among medical students: A two-site randomized controlled study *Journal of Psychosomatic Research*. Dec;

103: 102–7. https://doi.org/10.1016/j
.jpsychores.2017.10.008. Epub 2017 Oct 17.

General Medical Council (2015). Promoting
excellence: Standards for medical education
and training. Code GMC/PE/0715 (London,
United Kingdom).

Torppa, M. A., Makkohen, E., Mårtenson, C.,
and Pitkälä, K. H. (2008). A qualitative
analysis of student Balint groups in medical
education: Contexts and triggers of case
presentations and discussion themes. *Patient
Education and Counselling.* Jul; **72** (1): 5–11.
https://doi.org/10.1016/j.pec.2008.01.012.
Epub 2008 Mar 4.

Yazdankhahfard, M., Haghani, F., and Omid, A
(2019). The Balint group and its application
in medical education: A systematic review.
Journal of Education and Health Promotion.
8: 124.

Further Online Resources

More information about Balint groups is
available on the UK Balint Society website
http://balint.co.uk/, including a short video
made by medical students from Sheffield
University (https://balint.co.uk/medical-
students/).

Internationally, the Balint Society of
Australia and New Zealand and the
American Balint Society websites also
provide a wealth of information: www
.balintaustralianewzealand.org/; https://
americanbalintsociety.org/.

Teaching the Mental State Examination: An Example of Multimodal Teaching

4.7

Dr Patrick Hughes

Introduction

This chapter will explore how a teaching session focussed on mental state examination was redesigned for Year 3 medical students. Some of the pedagogical considerations that underpinned the redesign of the teaching session will be explored. Finally, the importance of embedding an evaluation process into the session will be discussed.

Context

The University of Glasgow has an existing undergraduate medical curriculum incorporating many of the professional competencies outlined in the GMC's Outcomes for Graduates (2018). The curriculum is comprised of Intended Learning Outcomes (ILOs), which in turn are grouped into three domains: knowledge, skills, and behaviours. The mental state examination (MSE) is an essential clinical skill for all doctors and medical students and so is represented in the curriculum as shown in Table 4.7.1.

Historically, the MSE session was taught in the form of a didactic lecture in Year 3. Given the nature of the learning material and the need to develop skills and behaviour, it was recognised that the format of this session required review.

Due to the need to incorporate opportunities to develop clinical skills and explore attitudes, a decision was made to redesign the session to provide better opportunities for learning and practice. The redesign of the session was underpinned by a number of pedagogical principles.

Planning

To develop and deliver the content of the new MSE session, a small group of clinicians and academics was formed to lead the teaching review. This group consisted of the undergraduate psychiatric teaching lead, a clinical academic experienced in teaching, and a higher trainee in psychiatry.

The ILOs for the session were reviewed and the initial discussion focussed on which teaching format(s) would be best to meet the ILOs and the learning needs of the students. This had to be balanced against both what was practically possible in the time frame given and the large number of students (around 300) that were required to attend the session over a two-day period.

While there were clearly facts to be learnt and concepts to be understood – types of knowledge that could be easily delivered through a lecture – it was also clear that students would need an opportunity to practise the clinical skills that required development. Small group teaching – and role play specifically – can provide students with an opportunity to

Table 4.7.1 Mental state examination: knowledge, skills and behaviour

Mental State Examination	Knowledge	Understand the components of mental state examination. Understand the basis for clinical signs on mental state examination and the relevance of positive and negative findings.
	Skills	Perform a detailed mental state examination, relevant to the presentation and risk factors, that is valid, targeted and time efficient. Interpret findings from the history, physical examination, and mental state examination, appreciating the importance of clinical, psychological, religious, social, and cultural factors.
	Behaviour	Show respect and behave in accordance with Good Medical Practice.

develop skills in a safe, controlled environment while providing learning support to help link the theory with practice. This type of teaching can also allow attitudes and beliefs to be explored, which forms an important part of the professionalism described in the final ILO.

Resources

Having identified that a multimodal approach would be undertaken, the existing resources were reviewed and scrutinised. Resources such as money, availability of facilitators, physical space, timetabling, physical equipment, pre-existing learning material, IT resources, and use of actors were all considered.

As there was no additional budget available for the session there was no scope to pay actors to act as simulated patients. While the university employs a small number of psychiatrists in research and teaching roles, there were not enough to facilitate small group teaching sessions for 300 students. However, it was noted that a large untapped resource available locally was that of Core and Higher Psychiatric trainees who are required to develop teaching competencies as part of their own postgraduate curriculum. This training requirement is most often met through local teaching, with little opportunity for trainees to get involved in formal undergraduate education at the university. The teaching review group hypothesised that recruiting these trainees as facilitators for the session could have a positive impact on both the undergraduate students and the trainees themselves by promoting near-peer learning and promoting the visibility of psychiatry in the curriculum.

As shown in Chapter 4.2, Nisha Dogra and Khalid Kalim advise that groups of between 8 and 12 students are most effective for small group teaching. Given there were approximately 300 students, this meant organising at least 25 rooms, with 25 trainees to act as facilitators. As there was neither the physical space nor enough trainees to do this, we decided to split the year into four cohorts who would each attend a three-hour session over four half-days. This meant that a smaller space would be required, and some facilitators would be able to participate in more than one session depending on availability.

To facilitate the small group teaching it was recognised that a computer, projector, speakers, and chairs would be required for each room.

Lesson Plan

Before the Small Group Teaching Session, the 'Flipped Classroom'

A 'flipped classroom' approach was adopted, and students were asked to watch a recorded PowerPoint presentation on the MSE in advance. Chapter 5.2 describes how this technique can allow knowledge and comprehension to occur outside the class, permitting the teacher to focus on higher-order skills during the session (Brame, 2013).

This pre-recorded lecture introduced the structure and key concepts of the MSE, and also described the relevant psychopathology to look for while undertaking the MSE. The pre-recorded material was available on the university's virtual learning platform several weeks before the small group session was due to take place. Students were advised to watch this lecture and familiarise themselves with the learning material ahead of their small group teaching session.

The Small Group Teaching Session

The three-hour small group teaching session was organised into eight twenty-minute blocks of teaching, with a break after four blocks of teaching activity.

Students were divided into small groups of between eight and twelve ahead of the session and were allocated to one of seven adjacent rooms within the medical school. The first twenty minutes were devoted to a brief recap of the 'flipped classroom' lecture, highlighting the key components of the MSE. This activated existing knowledge ahead of the practical part of the session but also provided some orientation and context for the students who hadn't watched the pre-recorded lecture beforehand.

After the recap session, the MSE teaching was divided into seven focussed interactive practical sessions, roughly aligned to the headings used in the standard MSE structure:

- Appearance, Behaviour, and Speech
- Mood and Affect
- Thought Form
- Thought Content
- Perception
- Cognition
- Insight and Judgement

One facilitator was allocated to each of these topics, and they delivered a focussed twenty-minute interactive session before moving onto the next group. Although this meant that the session ran for eighty minutes before the first break, we proposed that a different facilitator, teaching a different topic, using different methods every twenty minutes would serve to hold the students' attention better than sitting for the same length of time in a lecture.

The format of each interactive session varied depending on the topic. For example, the sessions on Appearance, Behaviour and Speech and Thought Form were tutorial based, incorporating video content of simulated patients during which students were asked to observe and make notes under several headings. The other sessions (e.g. Mood and Affect), incorporated opportunities for role play. As the students were largely unfamiliar with the MSE this was done in a very structured manner, with students being prepared with what kind of information they want to learn and what questions they might ask, prior to the facilitator assuming the role of the patient and being interviewed by one or more of the students.

Student Feedback and Quality Improvement

Given that a new multimodal teaching session had been developed, the teaching review panel recognised that it was important to obtain student and facilitator feedback to inform its improvement moving forward. As discussed in Chapter 6.3, student feedback can be a powerful mechanism for improving the learning experience (Fullana et al., 2016; Biwer et al., 2020; Deeley et al., 2019).

In this case, we opted to use an online survey to collect feedback from our students. This is a quick and easy way to gather views from a large number of students, but it has a number of limitations, especially when attempting to solicit feedback on a new teaching session. However, limited time and resources meant that, pragmatically, this was the most appropriate technique to use. The survey included Likert scales as well as open questions on what was good and what could be done better.

The feedback was examined, and the following changes were made to the session:

- The session was brought forward by several months to a more relevant part of the curriculum, having initially been delivered close to an important written exam on an unrelated topic.
- The content was reduced as it was felt to be too much to cover in the limited time available.
- The focus of the session was streamlined. Some of the theory was removed and put online, along with more of the psychopathology. The revised sessions were then more focussed on providing scaffolding to allow the inexperienced students to try the MSE in a controlled way.

The session has been delivered several times now and a process of gathering feedback and quality improvement is embedded within it, meaning that the session is continually being refined and improved to meet the learners' needs.

Lived Experience Involvement to Augment the Teaching Model

Gordon Johnston

One possible addition to this teaching model would be for people with lived experience to deliver some of the practical sessions, either through pre-recorded videos or in person, to the small groups. The content could be based on their own experiences or formed into anonymised and more archetypal case studies. While this would involve additional preparation and planning, with many of the same resource issues as outlined earlier, there could also be significant benefits for students.

While role play or facilitation in the manner described here can effectively enable development of student skills, the relationship will always have an artificial aspect to it. Even in a short session with a person with lived experience the student will be required to interact in a different manner, learning behaviours involving respect and developing their listening skills. The exercise will also enable students to see their patients as people rather than as collections of symptoms, and to gain deeper understanding of the effects of mental ill health.

Direct lived experience involvement in the educational process is common in many disciplines and feedback is generally good, with students reflecting positively on the opportunity to learn from first-hand experiences.

Conclusion

This chapter has outlined the development and delivery of a new multimodal teaching session incorporating many of the topics and principles described in this book. It illustrates how you can plan and deliver effective and efficient teaching underpinned by evidence-based educational theory. It also illustrates that it is not always necessary to have access to vast resources or sophisticated technology to deliver quality teaching. If teaching is approached in a systematic way, from identifying the learning needs to reflecting on the learning strategies available, with a pragmatic review of resources available and a structured process for gathering feedback, appraising the session, and making improvements, effective multimodal teaching can be harnessed to improve the educational experience of students and ultimately raise psychiatry's profile within undergraduate teaching.

References

Biwer, F., Oude Egbrink, M. G., Aalten, P., and de Bruin, A. B. (2020). Fostering effective learning strategies in higher education: A mixed-methods study. *Journal of Applied Research in Memory and Cognition*, **9** (2): 186–203.

Brame, C. (2013). Flipping the classroom. Vanderbilt University Center for Teaching. Retrieved 20 January 2021 from: http://cft.vanderbilt.edu/guides-sub-pages/flipping-the-classroom/Deeley, S. J.

Deeley, S. J., Fischbacher-Smith, M., Karadzhov, D., and Koristashevskaya, E. (2019). Exploring the 'wicked' problem of student dissatisfaction with assessment and feedback in higher education. *Higher Education Pedagogies*, **4** (1): 385–405.

Fullana, J., Pallisera, M., Colomer, J., et al. (2016). Reflective learning in higher education: A qualitative study on students' perceptions. *Studies in Higher Education*, **41** (6): 1008–22.

General Medical Council. (2018). *Outcomes for graduates* (online). Available at: www.gmc-uk.org/-/media/documents/outcomes-for-graduates-2020_pdf-84622587.pdf (accessed 20 January 2021).

Materials Development

Online Learning

Professor Jo-Anne Murray

Introduction

One benefit of the surge in technology is the development of online learning, which allows for the creation of engaging learning experiences for students to study what they want, where they want, and when they want. This is particularly relevant for online distance learners: for example, postgraduate trainees, who may also be juggling work and family alongside their studies.

However, technology has also been used to provide a blended learning experience for students, where a course includes both online and face-to-face (f2f) elements. Hybrid learning is very similar to blended learning in that a combination of online and f2f learning takes place, except in hybrid structures the focus is on finding a balance that promotes the best experience for individuals (Olapiriyakul and Scher, 2006). A further development is the hyflex model (Kyei-Blankson and Godwyll, 2010), whereby students are given the choice of whether to attend f2f or join the session online.

In psychiatry, there has been increased interest in online teaching and learning in recent years, which has developed further in response to the COVID-19 pandemic. Prior to COVID-19, however, medical students and trainees in psychiatry were already able to access significant amounts of learning materials online – more so, in fact, than printed materials. Moreover, much of the continual professional development (CPD) that has been provided in recent years has been delivered online, often by commercial CPD providers.

Online Learning Pedagogy

In recent times, there has been much discussion around the future of the f2f didactic lecture, with many predicting a move away from this and towards online and blended learning. Medical education has in many ways led the field in the move towards online learning, with a shift to incorporating online resources in undergraduate and postgraduate programmes. Moreover, the use of simulations has also been widely used in medical education, including psychiatry.

However, when designing or considering the use of online learning materials, it is important to consider the pedagogy of online learning. Pedagogy that is perceived as successful offline should be incorporated online (Alexander and Boud, 2001); however, this is not always the case. For example, what is considered as online learning is often little more than lectures delivered online in the form of text, audio, and/or video; indeed, uploading existing lectures to an online platform has been shown to cause students'/ participants' interest to quickly diminish (Bell et al., 2000), and that also includes uploading 'voice over presentations' that have been shown to overload attention (Mayer et al., 2001).

Thus, this approach is merely transmitting learning content without the interactivity of a lecturer who can promote discussion and answer questions. In psychiatry, learner outcomes appear to be optimised by a combination of didactic learning materials and interactive engagement, although too many modalities can be overwhelming to learners (Mankey, 2011). Alexander and Boud (2001) state that in online learning it is vital that learning designers 'provide activities to facilitate students' engaging with and making sense of content'. Thus, online learning is often defined as being based upon connectivism pedagogy. Connectivism pedagogy has been described as the process of building networks of information, contacts, and resources that are applied to real problems (Downes, 2007). Indeed, Warren et al. (2020) highlight the importance of conceptual understanding over surface learning, with that being at the forefront of consideration when designing online learning in psychiatry. In connectivism, learning begins when learners join together in a learning community, whereby the development of networks of both content and person can be applied to authentic problems (Strong and Hutchins, 2009). This has been described as a move from the age of the individual to the era of community (John-Steiner, 2006). Thus, online courses should be relevant, interactive, project-based, and collaborative, whilst providing leaners with some element of choice or control over the learning (Partlow and Gibbs, 2003). Using a scaffolding approach, wherein students are progressively moved towards greater independence and understanding, helps students to build on prior knowledge, form new associations, and achieve mastery (Warren et al., 2020). Such approaches emphasise the active role that learners play and are designed in such a way that learners can own' their learning and engage with topics that are personally meaningful (Shea et al., 2006). Another key consideration in designing online learning is ensuring clear signposting, both in terms of clarifying the core learning materials and activities that require completion and the additional resources provided, which is essential in ensuring that students do not become overwhelmed and reduce their focus on the key concepts that are necessary for them to learn (Mayer et al., 2001).

Pre-recorded lectures that can be paused, re-wound, and revisited can provide a foundation that can be built upon in increasing depth, and these can be augmented with case-based discussions on specific areas/topics and virtual patient simulations. Including branched decision-making elements into virtual patient simulations can enhance student engagement, cognitive processing, and problem solving (Schmidt et al., 2011). This branched design allows students to make decisions within the simulation and to experience the consequences of those decisions. Automated feedback can also be built into the scenarios to support learning. Case-based learning engages students in discussions of specific scenarios with real-world examples. This is a learner-centred approach that involves intense interactions between students as they develop their knowledge and work as a group to examine the case. In the traditional setting these conversations would typically take place face to face, but case-based discussions can also take place online. In fact, the concept of community for learning is of particular importance in online learning in general, and therefore educational practices should promote this form of communication between learners (Dawson, 2006).

Communication in Online Learning

Communication creates opportunities for learning to occur by clarifying information, promoting enthusiasm in learning, encouraging interaction, and building positive relationships between learners. Within the traditional classroom setting social and communicative interactions occur between student and teacher, and student and student (Picciano 2002). However, this face-to-face interaction cannot take place online where, instead interactions occur via the internet.

A lack of face-to-face interaction can impact on the learners' sense of belonging to a scholarly community (Rovai, 2002), resulting in students feeling isolated and insecure about their learning (Knapper, 1998), and even dropping out of their studies (Peters, 1992) Statistics show that 20–30% of students who begin a Distance Education (DE) course do not finish it (Rovai, 2002), and some suggest that programme retention rates are lower for online learning compared to their face-to-face counterparts (Russo and Campbell, 2004) This has been postulated to be due to online courses being less able to provide the personal interaction that students crave (Carr, 2000). Students studying online courses report feelings of social disconnectedness and missing the familiar teacher immediacy, interpersonal interactions, and social cues they more typically have when learning face-to-face if the design and delivery of the online course is not based on promoting communication and interaction (Slagter van Tron and Bishop, 2009). Therefore, whilst interaction is key in any educational setting, interaction in online courses is considered to be the cornerstone of effective pedagogical practices (Fulford and Zhang, 1993). By interacting, students can build a community of practice, wherein they engage in a process of collective learning. In medical education, including psychiatry, developing communities of practice can support learners with the complexity of the medical curricula (Cruess et al., 2018).

In medical education, including psychiatry teaching, there is a need to ensure that the richness of the face-to-face setting, where there is a guided discussion of topics/ideas, questioning of concepts, and an opportunity for self-reflection, is also captured/promoted online. However, a major challenge in medical education centres around discussing real cases. In face-to-face settings this takes place frequently as patients are more likely to give consent for in-person discussions, as compared to online settings due to the permanency and potential dissemination of online discussions (Hickey and McAleer, 2017). Another challenge is the use of clinical images in online learning in terms of the ethical implications which need to be considered and images used appropriately (Kornhaber et al., 2015). Nevertheless, online learning in psychiatry should incorporate mechanisms for good-quality and timely interactions, and there are various communication media that can be used to facilitate this.

Communication Media in Online Learning

Although technology does not implicitly improve learning, various communication media can be used in online learning to reduce the feelings of distance and isolation from peers and tutors, and to provide opportunities for collaborative learning activities (Bates, 2005). Technology has the ability to distort the concept of distance between learners and their instructor (Beldarrain, 2012). The twenty-first-century learner is someone who wants to stay connected to their peers, receive prompt feedback from their instructor, and prefers to work in a group setting rather than in isolation. However, technologies must be used in conjunction with appropriate pedagogical approaches; it is essential that pedagogy drives the use of technology, rather than the other way round (Beldarrain, 2012).

The more traditional communication media used in online learning include email and discussions boards within a Virtual Learning Environment (VLE). However, a new generation of communication media now exist, including social networking sites (e.g. Facebook and Twitter), instant messaging (e.g. WhatsApp and Microsoft Teams), virtual classrooms (e.g. Zoom), and virtual worlds (e.g. Second Life). The emergence of these new technologies provides opportunities for educators to foster interaction and collaboration between learners and build a learning community (Beldarrain, 2012). These tools can also promote social presence, which is important to consider in online learning. When social presence is lacking, people regard the environment as impersonal and consequently they share less and work less well together (Leh, 2001). Social presence has the ability to create warmth and support (Russo and Campbell, 2004), which can be difficult to do when using text-based means of communicating. Text-based communication can lack social presence due to a lack of non-verbal cues, such as facial expressions and gestures (Leh, 2001). In text-based communication the reader cannot access the sender's emotions unless the sender expresses them in the text. The use of social cues, such as smiles and encouraging gestures, is known to enhance learning (Hackman and Walker, 1990) and the absence of such cues in online can promote a less personal and less friendly approach to learning (Rice and Love, 1987). Emoticons can replace non-verbal cues (Gunawardena and Zittel, 1997), and it has been reported that well-developed interpersonal relationships can be formed online through text-based communication when emoticons are used (Walther, 1992).

Effective communication skills development (verbal and non-verbal) is of high importance in medical education and is an integral part of the medical curricula. The optimal approach to developing communication skills is considered to be by direct observation of the student's performance in a f2f setting followed by feedback from an experienced tutor (Smith et al., 2007). However, this is resource intensive and involves simulated patients and experienced tutors which, if there is a lack of standardisation of the patients or tutors, can result in unequal learning outcomes (Kyaw et al., 2019). In online learning, various approaches can be taken to develop communications skills – for example, using videos of simulated patient scenarios or virtual patients. The online platform can be used to deliver the theoretical concepts that underpin communication skills, and video simulations of patient scenarios can provide a demonstration of psychiatric assessment and mental state examination (Foster et al., 2014). The ability for students to annotate videos with notes can also further support their learning, and embedded quizzes can be helpful in tracking progress (Benjamin et al., 2006). Moreover, virtual patient simulations can be particularly useful where clinical scenarios are difficult to replicate with standardised patients, such as communication with patients that have rare conditions, speech disorders, and neurological diseases (Kyaw et al., 2019). Using online approaches allows students the flexibility to work through the scenarios as many times as required and can also be used to augment traditional face-to-face communications skills teaching. However, there are some aspects of communications skill, such as utilisation of empathy, that can be difficult to convey without face-to-face contact and observation (Hickey and McAleer, 2017). Therefore, using a blend of online and face-to-face teaching can be beneficial and also allows students to practise their skills interchangeably. Blended learning has been used in psychiatry teaching with promising outcomes, particularly the flipped classroom concept, whereby content is viewed online prior to face-to-face tutorials that are used to reinforce, integrate, develop, and apply knowledge (Prober and Heath, 2012).

Asynchronous and Synchronous Communication

Communication in online learning can be asynchronous or synchronous. Asynchronous technologies provide opportunities for instructor–student and student–student time-delayed collaboration. The most commonly used asynchronous technology is discussions boards within the VLE (Russo and Campbell, 2004). Asynchronous discussions boards can have multiple threads with several discussions and interactions progressing simultaneously. In this scenario, students can respond to the tutor and other students, and can initiate and respond to threads depending on their interests and points of view. Some students appear to prefer asynchronous communication since, in addition to the flexibility afforded by the 'anytime, anywhere' mode, this approach to communicating gives the learners time to reflect before responding. Time for reflection can reduce apprehension in those individuals that are more likely to withhold their ideas from fear of others not approving (Gallupe et al., 1992). This approach can also be advantageous to those who are reticent or have trouble articulating ideas, or who use English as a second language (Russo and Campbell, 2004). Online discussion boards can also allow students to access senior clinicians/tutors and diverse peer support beyond their friendship groups, and can facilitate deeper and more diverse discussions. These boards do have to be monitored, and clear guidance on use and etiquette should be provided that aligns with professional standards (Walter et al., 2004).

However, asynchronous communication can pose issues for some learners, whereby time-delayed responses may result in messages appearing out of context and hence being less meaningful, especially if a student has moved on to another topic or task (Russo and Campbell, 2004). They can also lack immediacy, which can limit some student's responses to other student's and instructor's comments (Childress and Braswell, 2006). Conversely, synchronous technologies allow students and instructors to interact in real-time despite being located remotely. Examples of synchronous technologies used in the delivery of online learning include web conferencing technologies for real-time interaction between course participants and virtual classrooms for presentation and discussion of learning materials in real time. Web-conferencing technologies (such as Skype) offer real-time text-based or audio discussions, whilst virtual classrooms (e.g. Zoom) provide live features such as audio, video, application sharing, and content display to support synchronous collaboration (De Lucia et al., 2009). Moreover, virtual worlds (such as Second Life) may provide an additional level of interaction that can be absent in other collaborative media by providing an interactive 3D environment, avatars that act as visual representations of users, and an interactive chat (and often audio) tool for users to communicate with each other (Murray et al., 2015). Indeed, virtual worlds have been used in medical education for simulation of clinical setting and procedures (Wiecha et al., 2010), and have also been used for role play simulation in psychiatry (Vallance et al., 2014).

Such technologies can provide just-in-time clarification and information (Simkins et al., 2009), and learners can receive an immediate recognition of their efforts and contribution to the course which, in turn, encourages autonomous and active learning.

Lived Experience Involvement in Online Learning

Gordon Johnston

The involvement of people with lived experience can be successfully introduced into online learning if carefully planned and facilitated. For some people, giving a presentation or talk remotely using Zoom or Teams may be easier than facing a live audience, especially when discussing personal or highly emotive (and therefore potentially triggering) episodes from their own past. For others, their preferred method may be to record a video.

It is important to discuss and agree potential methods of delivery with those to be involved as early as possible. This facilitates good planning, allows adequate time for preparation, and also reduces anxiety by ensuring good understanding of exactly what they are agreeing to do.

Assuming appropriate technologies are available, people with lived experience can contribute effectively to remote or blended learning environments in a variety of ways. Finding the best method to enable them to do so while also feeling safe and supported is key to success.

Considerations

Online learning provides many benefits and opportunities; however, there are some key areas that need to be considered. Developing content for online delivery is time consuming and requires careful planning and consideration. There also needs to be buy-in from the institution to support a move to online, which includes resources: the technology itself, support to use the technology, and recognition of the time it takes to develop the online learning materials.

Not all teaching staff may be confident or enthusiastic about teaching online and therefore support for staff developing online learning materials is an important consideration. Clinicians are very busy and thus have little time to learn new technologies. Furthermore, it is important not to lose the input of an experienced clinician to whom the prospect of teaching online is daunting. It cannot be assumed that all students are digitally literate or have access to technology and the Internet. Internet speed and bandwidth may also be inconsistent across student cohorts depending on their location, which can affect access to videos or downloading content. Also, content needs to be accessible on many devices, such as PCs, laptops, and smart phones. Students may also need support to develop their digital literacies and to become successful online learners. Digital professionalism needs to be built into the curricula.

Conclusion

Online learning continues to increase in use in all education sectors, including medical education and psychiatry teaching. Online learning in psychiatry can be used as a blended approach whereby online and face-to-face approaches are synergistic. This can be especially helpful for geographically diverse locations. Online learning can foster community building and the development of a community of practice. Online simulations offer the opportunity for students to experience the consequences of their decision making in case-based scenarios. There are many benefits and opportunities provided by online learning; however, planning, time, and commitment are required to deliver an effective learning experience online.

References

Alexander, S. and Boud, D. (2001). Learners still learn from experience when online. In J. Stephenson (ed.) *Teaching and Learning Online: Pedagogies for New Technologies*, pp. 3–15. London: Kogan Page.

Bates, A. W. (2005). *Technology, E-learning and Distance Education*. London: Routledge.

Beldarrain, Y. (2012). Distance education trends: Integrating new technologies to foster student interaction and collaboration. *Distance Education*, 27 (2): 139–53.

Bell, D. S., Fanarow, G. C. and Hays, R. D. (2000). Self-study from web-based and printed guided materials. A randomised, controlled trial among resident physicians. *Annals of Internal Medicine*, **132**, 938–46.

Benjamin, S., Robbins, L. I., Kung, S. (2006). Online resources for assessment and evaluation. *Academic Psychiatry*, **30**, 498–504.

Carr, S. (2000). As distance education comes of age, the challenge is keeping the students. *Chronicle of Higher Education*, **46** (23): A39–A41.

Childress, M. D. and Braswell, R. (2006). Using massively multiplayer online role-playing games for online learning. *Distance Education*, 27 (2): 187–96.

Cruess, R. L., Cruess, S. R., and Steinert, Y. (2018). Medicine and a community of practice: Implications for medical education. *Academic Medicine*, **93** (2): 185–91.

Dawson, S. (2006). A study of the relationship between student communication interaction and sense of community. *The Internet and Higher Education*, **9** (3): 153–62.

De Lucia, A., Francese, R., Passero, I., and Tortora, G. (2009). Development and evaluation of a virtual campus on Second Life: The case of SecondDMI. *Computers and Education*, **52** (1): 220–33.

Downes, W. (2007). An introduction to connective knowledge. *International Conference on Media, Knowledge and Education – exploring new spaces, relations and dynamics in digital media ecologies* (online). https://www.downes.ca/post/33034 (accessed 30 July 2020).

Foster, A., Johnson, T., Liu, H. et al. (2014). Psychiatry clinical simulation online teaching modules: A multi-site prospective study of student assessments. *MedEdPublish*, 3, 30.

Fulford, C. P. and Zhang, S. (1993). Perceptions of interactions: The critical predictor in distance education. *Distance Education*, 7, 8–21.

Gallupe, R. B., Dennis, A. R., Cooper, W. H., et al. (1992). Electronic brainstorming and group size. *The Academy of Management Journal*, **35** (2): 350–69. https://doi.org/10.2307/256377.

Gunawardena, C. and Zittel, F. (1997). Social presence as a predictor of satisfaction within a computermediated conferencing environment. *The American Journal of Distance Education*, **11** (3): 8–26.

Hackman, M. Z. and Walker, K. B. (1990). Instructional communication in the televised classroom: The effects of system design and teacher immediacy on student learning and satisfaction. *Communication Education*, **39** (3): 196–209.

Hickey, C. M. and McAleer, S. (2017). Designing and developing an online module: A 10-step approach. *Academic Psychiatry*, **41**, 106–9.

John-Steiner, V. (2006). *Creative collaborations*. New York: Oxford University Press.

Knapper, C. K. (1988). Lifelong learning and distance education. *American Journal of Distance Education*, **2** (1): 63–72. Available at: www.learntechlib.org/p/139170/ (accessed 27 March 2022).

Kornhaber, R., Betihavas, V., and Baber, R. J. (2015). Ethical implications of digital images for teaching and learning purposes: An integrative review. *Journal of Multidisciplinary Healthcare*, **8**, 299–305.

Kyaw, B. M., Posadzki, P., Paddock, S., et al. (2019). Effectiveness of digital education on communication skills among medical students: Systematic review and meta-analysis by the digital health collaboration. *Journal of Medical Internet Research*, **21** (8). Available at: www.jmir.org/2019/8/e12967/?amp;utm_medium=twitter#Introduction (accessed 30 October 2020).

Kyei-Blankson, L. and Godwyll, F. (2010). An examination of learning outcomes in hyflex learning environments. *The Learning Technology Library* (online). Available at: www.learntechlib.org/p/35598/ (accessed 30 July 2020).

Leh, A. S. (2001). Computer-mediated communication and social presence in a distance learning environment.

International Journal of Educational Telecommunications, **7** (2): 109–28.

Mankey, V. L. (2011). Using multimodal and multimedia tools in the psychiatric education of diverse learners: Examples from the mental status exam. *Academic Psychiatry*, **35**, 335–9.

Mayer, R. E., Heiser, J., and Lonn, S. (2001). Cognitive constraints on multimedia learning: when presenting more materials results in less understanding. *Journal of Educational Psychology*, **93**, 187.

Murray, J. M. D., Hale, F., and Dozier, M. (2015). Use and perception of Second Life by distance learners: Comparison with other communication media. *International Journal of E-learning and Distance Education*, **30** (2).

Olapiriyakul, K. and Scher, J. M. (2006). A guide to establishing hybrid learning courses: Employing information technology to create a new learning experience, and a case study. *The Internet and Higher Education*, **3** (4): 287–301.

Partlow, K. M. and Gibbs, W. J. (2003). Indicators of constructivist principles in internet-based courses. *J. Comput. High. Educ.* **14** (68). https://doi.org/10.1007/BF02940939.

Peters, O. (1992). Some observations on dropping out in distance education. *Distance Education*, **13**: 234–69.

Picciano, A. G. (2002). Beyond student perceptions: Issues of interaction, presence, and performance in an online course. *Journal of Asynchronous Learning Network*, **6** (1): 21–40.

Prober, C. G. and Heath, C. (2012). Lecture halls without lectures – a proposal for medical education. *New England Journal of Medicine*, **366**, 1657–9.

Rovai, A. (2002). Building a sense of community at a distance. *The International Review of Open and Distributed Learning*, **3** (1): 1–16.

Russo, T. C. and Campbell, S. W. (2004). Perceptions of mediated presence in an asynchronous online course: Interplay of communication behaviours and medium. *Distance Education*, **25** (2): 215–32.

Schmidt, H. G., Rotgans, J. I., Yew, E. H. J. (2011). The process of problem-based learning: What works and why. *Medical Education*, **45**, 792–806.

Shea, P., Sau, L. C., and Pickett, A. (2006). A study of teaching presence and student sense of learning community in fully online and web-enhanced college courses. *The Internet and Higher Education*, **9** (3): 175–90.

Simkins, S., Maier, M., and Rhem, J. (2009). *Just-In-Time Teaching: Across the Disciplines, and Across the Academy (New Pedagogies and Practices for Teaching in Higher Education)*. Virginia: Stylus Publishing.

Slagter van Tron, P. J. and Bishop, M. J. (2009). Theoretical foundations for enhancing social connectedness in online learning environments. *Distance Education*, **30** (3): 291–315.

Smith, S., Hanson, J. L., Tewksbury, L. R., et al. (2007). Teaching patient communication skills to medical students: A review of randomized controlled trials. *Evaluation and the Health Professions*, **30** (1): 3–21.

Strong, K. and Hutchins, H. M. (2009). Connectivism: A theory for learning in a world of growing complexity. *Journal of Applied Research in Workplace E-Learning*, **1** (1): 53–67.

Vallance, A. K., Hemani, A., Fernandez, V., and Livingstone. D. (2014). Using virtual worlds for role play simulation in child and adolescent psychiatry: An evaluation study. *The Psychiatric Bulletin*, **8** (5): 204–10.

Walter, D. A., Rosenquist, P. B., and Bawtinhimer, G. (2004). Distance learning technologies in the training of psychiatry residents: A critical assessment. *Academic Psychiatry*, **28**, 60–5.

Walther, J. B. (1992). Interpersonal effects in computer-mediated interaction: A relational perspective. *Communication Research*, **19**, 52–90.

Warren, N., Parker, S., Khoo, T., Cabral, S., and Turner, J. (2020). Challenges and solutions when developing online interactive psychiatric education. *Australasian Psychiatry*, **28** (3): 359–62. https://doi.org/10.1177/1039856220901477.

Wiecha, J., Heyden, R., Sternthal, E., and Merialdi, M. (2010). Learning in a virtual world: Experience with using second life for medical education. *Journal of Medical Internet Research*. **12**. e1. 10.2196/jmir.1337.

The Flipped Classroom

Laura McNaughton and Neeraj Bhardwaj

The 'flipped classroom' is an active learning approach which has been adopted by many teaching professionals across educational institutes. There is much debate around the origins of the flipped classroom; however, many give credit to Jonathan Bergmann and Aaron Sams for bringing the approach to popular attention. They 'flipped' their classroom in 2007 with the use of pre-recorded content. In the early 2000s, Salman Khan also 'flipped' his classroom with the use of pre-recorded instructional video lectures, which later led to the formation of the Khan Academy (2004). Today, the Khan Academy, Coursera, TED (Technology, Entertainment and Design) talks, and even YouTube are online resources associated with the flipped classroom.

Now more than ever, medical schools are being challenged 'to better prepare their students to meet the evolving healthcare needs of society' (McLaughlin et al., 2014, p. 236). Due to the ever-growing need for enhanced skills, education has seen increased awareness in the use of active learning methods to 'engage learners and promote knowledge application over knowledge acquisition' (Sandrone et al., 2020).

Furthermore, the global COVID-19 pandemic has led to a shift in all educational institutes towards an increased awareness and acceptance 'of the innovative potential that technology, including emergent technology, can offer to enhance teaching and learning across the continuum of medical education' (Goh, 2020, p. 4). This chapter will explore what the flipped classroom is, how the flipped classroom approach can be embedded, and considerations for successful implementation.

What Exactly is a Flipped Classroom?

The flipped classroom is, in essence, an 'inverted' or 'reversed' classroom. What we mean by this is that the traditional classroom approach of sharing knowledge together simultaneously in a room is 'inverted' so that the uptake of knowledge – in the form of learning materials, such as pre-recorded video lectures – is completed at the learner's own pace prior to attending the class. This 'flips' the traditional activities conducted in the classroom (e.g. lectures) with at home tasks (i.e. problem-based activities, group work) (Lawson, Davis, and Son, 2019; Comber and Brady-Van den Bos, 2018; Hwang, Lai, and Wang, 2015; Lage, Platt, and Treglia, 2000).

A flipped classroom, in theory, allows learners to progress to a higher level of the cognitive processes discussed in Bloom's revised taxonomy (2001) (Lawson, Davis, and Son, 2019; Burke and Fedorek, 2017; Bergmann and Sams, 2012). The lower levels of cognitive processes – gaining knowledge and comprehension – take place outside of class, focussing on the higher forms of cognitive process – application, analysis, synthesis, and evaluation – during class (Brame, 2013).

Table 5.2.1 Advantages and disadvantages of the flipped classroom

Advantages

o Encourages **self-determination** and can **reduce cognitive load,** because class time is structured to inspire learners to be more 'active participants', facilitating 'autonomy and competence' (Abeysekera and Dawson, 2014, p. 5)

o 'Learning-centred model' (Burke and Fedorek 2017, p. 12; Roehl et al., 2013)

o Space for learners to 'take **responsibility for their own learning**' (Bergmann, Overmyer, and Wilie, 2011, p. 3)

o Educators can more easily alter their approach to meet the needs of learners with learning difficulties, as **self-paced** 'mastery learning' provides learners with **choice in how they build understanding** through learning content (Altemueller and Lindquist, 2017 p. 341)

Disadvantages

o The flipped classroom is based on **the foundation that learners arrive to class prepared**; however this is not always the case, and is considered one of the biggest barriers to the effectiveness of this approach (Burke and Fedorek, 2017; Bristol, 2014; Kim et al., 2014; Ebbeler, 2013)

o A **lack of access** (e.g. devices or materials), **skills, or attitudes** will 'undermine autonomy' creating dissatisfaction with the learning experience, thereby emphasising the importance of the educator's role in leading the flipped classroom approach (Adekola, Dale, and Gardiner, 2017)

Table 5.2.1 summarises the advantages and disadvantages of using a flipped approach.

Current research suggests that the flipped classroom approach in health education can lead to a significant improvement in student learning when compared with traditional teaching methods (Hew and Lo, 2018). Låg and Sæle (2019) undertook an in-depth meta-analysis of 271 sample studies which highlighted that, on average, student learning – measured by exam scores, test scores, or grades – was often more than one-fifth of a standard deviation higher under flipped conditions than in traditional classrooms. Furthermore, Freeman et al. (2014) conducted a meta-analysis of 225 studies in undergraduate courses highlighting active learning approaches, such as the flipped classroom, as students' preferred teaching and learning method. Despite this, research into the development of 'evidence-based guidelines' for flipped classroom implementation is limited (Khanova et al., 2015).

A Flipping Success? Embedding the Flipped Approach

The method of flipping a class is often associated with the mistaken belief that it requires 'merely an inversion' of the activities that occur in and outside of the classroom (Isaias, 2018, p. 141). However flipping a class, or indeed a full course, requires planning and knowledge of the demands and effort it entails.

The essential actions for implementing a flipped classroom are:

Before 'Class'

The first step in embedding the flipped classroom approach is that of building 'incentive' (Lam, Lau, and Chan, 2019; Brame, 2013) through clear setting of expectations and standards for students. This is essential as it is important that the students understand the

---

Box 5.2.1 Tips for Flipping the Classroom Before Class

To do …

- Clearly explain approach and expectations – **Incentive**
- Set goals (What are the course learning outcomes?) – **Incentive**
- Develop learning materials (e.g. lectures, e-Learning, video case studies, etc.) – **Exposure**
- Assign pre-class tasks (e.g. group work, discussion forums, reading list, case study analysis, data collection, etc.) – **Exposure**
- Design activities (group work, practical, discussion, etc.) – **Activities**

---

aim of this approach and how it will work, and that they are aware of their new responsibilities in maintaining satisfactory involvement in their courses (Isaias, 2018; Miles and Foggett, 2016). Additionally, to help prepare students for the transition from traditional methods of teaching to the flipped approach, explaining the benefits of this approach to students can ease anxiety and concern (Sezer and Abay, 2019).

The amount of time required to prepare for a class session is a common concern for learners, while the lack of preparation time for developing materials is a source of apprehension for educators (Sandrone et al., 2020). Educators should ensure that the workload of their students is evenly balanced between pre-class and in-class and not expanded, and that students are aware of the time input required at each stage (Isaias, 2018; Loveys et al., 2016).

Educators should initially limit the number of content topics, which will allow learners increased time to adapt to this new pedagogical approach (Isaias, 2018). In addition, initial 'exposure' materials should focus on how to use available learning resources and the associated technologies, along with when and why specific tools are best utilised, in order to support students in identifying how they can achieve academic success (Miles and Foggett, 2016). Learning materials associated with a successful flipped approach are described as 'edited, concise, simple and engaging', and it is noted that an 'unmanageable volume of pre-class learning materials' can lead to students coming to class under prepared to participate (Khanova et al., 2015, pp. 1042, 1045). Research highlights that it is essential that learning materials, particularly lecture content, is available for students to review and re-review as required (Isaias, 2018; Kim et al., 2014).

Learning activities, both pre-class and in-class, should be designed to closely align with course learning outcomes and clearly identify the purpose of the activity for students (Låg and Sæle, 2019). Bergmann and Sams (2013) suggest that the flipped approach should begin with one simple question: what is the best use of your class time?

During 'Class'

In this stage of the flipped classroom, educators create space to allow their students to practice (activities) the knowledge they have gained through learning materials (exposure), while assessing knowledge assimilation (assess) and providing encouragement and reward through praise (incentive) for higher-level thinking (Lam, Lau, and Chan, 2019; Brame, 2013).

Educators must ensure that their students are aware of the 'explicit connections' between the learning materials, activities, and overall goal of the class (Lawson, Davis, and Son, 2019).

> **Box 5.2.2 Tips for Flipping the Classroom During Class**
>
> **To do ...**
>
> - Offer support to students, review content to help students assess their own knowledge and skills – **Assess**
> - Assess students through in class activities (quizzes, discussions, practical, etc.) – **Assess**
> - Help students to focus on the content of learning through facilitation of in-class activities – **Activities**
> - Give scores as incentives – **Incentives**

In addition, educators require the confidence that their students, upon arrival in class, have learnt the necessary information and skills from completion of learning materials to participate in learning activities (Jensen et al., 2018). Research suggests that the simplest way to gauge student preparedness is via quizzes or formative assessment, conducted through pre-class tasks and at the beginning of in-class sessions. Quizzes at the start of a class can make the class more efficient, as these quizzes help students to recall the knowledge learnt in pre-class materials and hence participate productively in activities (Hew and Lo, 2018).

Another aspect of a successful flipped classroom is that of building an environment in class that supports students to develop ideas and knowledge application through use of contextually real situations during activities (Logan, 2015). Discussion tasks, set both in-class and out of class as forums, can be a useful tool in creating space to allow students to contextualise the knowledge gained. For discussions to be effective they must be structured to visibly identify the purpose and expectations of participation while encouraging students to co-create expertise (Chen et al., 2017).

In terms of support, well-timed constructive responses from educators have a big impact on student participation and successful implementation of the flipped approach. Martin, Wang, and Sadaf (2018) highlighted that well-timed responses to email and discussion forums, quick turnaround of educator grading and feedback on assessments, and effective educator response to student contributions appeared to be significantly influential on key outcomes.

After 'Class'

The key areas for consideration in the final stages of the flipped approach centre around educator support (incentive), assessments that evaluate students' understanding of the material (assess), and collaboration (activities) (Brame, 2013).

Effective support from the educator, as highlighted previously, is an essential component of the flipped approach, in particular immediate constructive feedback and suggestions for how students can make improvements for success (Young and Nichols, 2017). Timely feedback can support students to refine their time management practices, along with the ability to revisit activities, learning materials, and discussions (Uzir et al., 2019).

Another key aspect is that of creating space to allow students to mentor and collaborate with each other (Logan, 2015). Research conducted by Kim et al. (2014) highlights the importance of developing a learning community, through facilitation of student collaborations, in the flipped approach. In order to do this, appropriate communication channels should be created to allow students to interact with their peers and the educator (Isaias, 2018).

Finally, in terms of summative assessment in the flipped approach, it is essential that assessments are aligned with the learning outcomes that were clearly explained at the beginning of the course and the learning activities that take place during class (Sharma et al., 2015). Additionally, assessments need to be structured to allow students to demonstrate the higher-order thinking skills, discussed in Bloom's Taxonomy (2001), that they have developed through participation in the flipped approach.

This model (Figure 5.2.1) summarises the key considerations and essential actions for implementing a successful flipped classroom approach.

Box 5.2.3 Tips for Flipping the Classroom After Class

To do . . .

- Offer additional support to students – **Incentive**
- Allow space for students to collaborate and coach each other – **Exposure**
- Highlight areas of best practice, giving praise to students who have excelled in these areas – **Incentive**
- Design assessments connected to pre-class tasks, in-class activities, and core learning outcomes – **Assess, Activities**

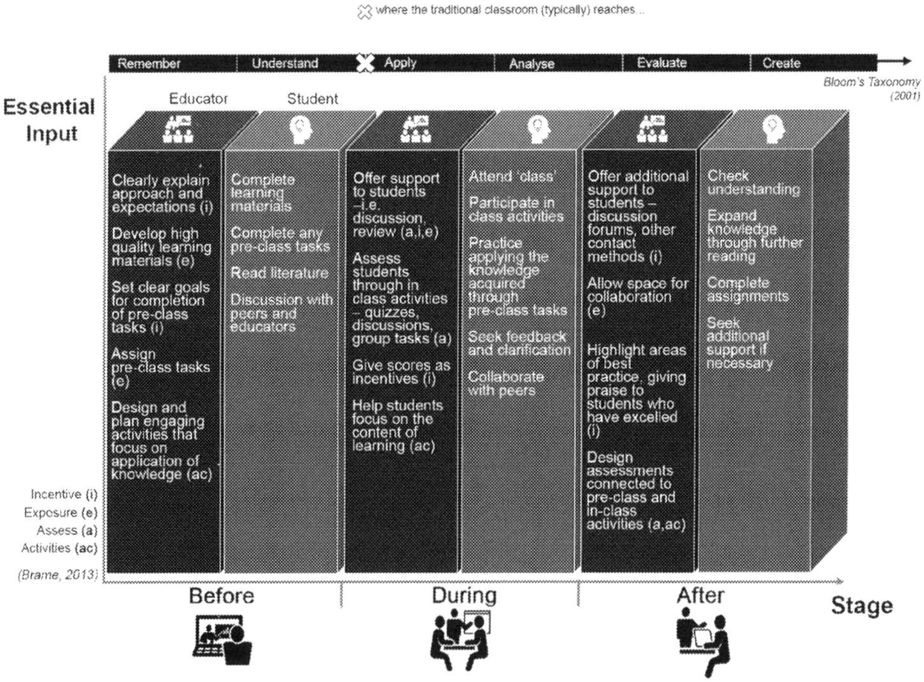

Figure 5.2.1 Key considerations and essential actions for successfully flipping the classroom

Let's Flip It . . .

In conclusion, the flipped classroom approach, when delivered effectively, has the possibility to better prepare students for the evolving workplace of today, through creating a learning environment which allows the development of higher-order thinking (Sandrone et al., 2020).

In order to successfully embed the flipped approach, educators need to be mindful of the change in roles and input required and the time and effort needed to develop motivation (incentive), learning materials (exposure), activities, assessments (assess), and impactful support mechanisms (Brame, 2013).

Overall, to ensure successful implementation it is key that educators consider the crucial pedagogical components: the need to 'conceptualise' new methods and models of learning and teaching, to highlight the needs and expectations of students, and to build strong alignment of assessments with the course learning outcomes and activities that address these learner needs (Adekola, Dale, and Gardiner, 2017).

When considering future flipped classroom approaches, educators should be mindful of potential external factors, such as the COVID-19 pandemic that resulted in a global shift of awareness and acceptance in online learning and the importance of technologies, particularly emerging technologies, as a support mechanism for leaners (Sandrone et al., 2020; Shah and Barkas, 2018).

References

Abeysekera, L. and Dawson, P. (2014). Motivation and cognitive load in the flipped classroom: Definition, rationale and a call for research. *Higher Education Research & Development*, **34** (1): 1–14.

Adekola, J., Dale, V. H. M., and Gardiner, K. (2017). Development of an institutional framework to guide transitions into enhanced blended learning in higher education. Learning Enhancement and Academic Development Service, University of Glasgow. *ALT: Research in Learning Technology 2017*, **25**: http://dx.doi.org/10.25304/rlt.v25.1973 (accessed May 2020).

Adekola, J., Dale, V. H. M., Gardiner, K., and Fischbacher-smith, M. (2017). Student transitions to blended learning: An institutional case study. *Journal of Perspectives in Applied Academic Practice*, **5** (2): 58–65.

Akçayır, G. and Akçayır, M. (2018). The flipped classroom: a review of its advantages and challenges. *Computer and Education*, **126**, 334–45.

Altemueller, L. and Lindquist, C. (2017). Flipped classroom instruction for inclusive learning. *British Journal of Special Education*, **44** (3).

Arnold-Garza, S. (2014). The Flipped Classroom Teaching Model and its use for Information Literacy Instruction. *Communication in Information Literacy*, **8**.

Bergmann, J., Overmyer, J., and Wilie, B. (2011). The flipped class: Myths vs. reality. https://doi.org/10.1037/00220663.81.3.329. Available at: https://kmtrosclair.files.wordpress.com/2015/06/the-flipped-class-myths-vs-reality-the-daily-riff-be-smarter-about-education.pdf (accessed April 2020).

Bergmann, J. and Sams, A. (2012). *Flip your classroom: How to reach every student in every class every day*. Washington, DC: International Society for Technology in Education.

Bloom, B. S., Anderson, L. W., and Krathwohl, D. (2001). *A Taxonomy for Learning, Teaching, and Assessing: A Revision of Bloom's Taxonomy of Educational Objectives*. Longman.

Brame, C. (2013). Flipping the classroom. Vanderbilt University Center for Teaching. Retrieved 1 June 2020 from http://cft.vanderbilt.edu/guides-sub-pages/flipping-the-classroom/.

Bristol, T. J. (2014). Flipping the classroom. *Teaching and Learning in Nursing*, **9** (1): 43–6.

Burke, A. S. and Fedorek, B. (2017). Does 'flipping' promote engagement?: A comparison of a traditional, online, and flipped class. *Active Learning in Higher Education*, **18** (1): 11–24. https://doi.org/10.1177/1469787417693487 (accessed May 2020).

Chen, B., deNoyelles, A., Patton, K., and Zydney, J. (2017). Creating a community of inquiry in large-enrollment online courses: An exploratory study on the effect of protocols within online discussions. *Online Learning*, **21** (1): 165–88.

Chen, C. M. and Wu, C. H. (2015). Effects of different video lecture types on sustained attention, emotion, cognitive load, and learning performance. *Computers & Education*, **80**. 108–21.

Comber, D. P. M. and Brady-Van den Bos, M. (2018). Too much, too soon? A critical investigation into factors that make Flipped Classrooms effective. *Higher Education. Research & Development*, 37:4, 683–97.

Demski, J. (2013). 6 Expert Tips for Flipping the Classroom. *Tech-enabled Learning*. Online blog, available at: https://campustechnology.com/articles/2013/01/23/6-expert-tips-for-flipping-the-classroom.aspx (accessed June 2020).

Ebbeler, J. (2013). '"Introduction to Ancient Rome", the flipped version'. *The Chronicle of Higher Education*, 22 July. Available at: http://chronicle.com/article/Introduction-to-Ancient/140475/ (accessed 27 March 2022).

Freeman, S., Eddy, S. L., McDonough, M., et al. (2014). Active learning increases student performance in science, engineering, and mathematics. *Proc Natl Acad Sci*, **111**: 8410–5. https://doi.org/10.1073/pnas.1319030111.

Goh, P. S. (2016). eLearning or Technology enhanced learning in medical education – hope, not hype, *Medical Teacher*, **38** (9): 957–8. https://doi.org/10.3109/0142159X.2016.1147538.

Goh, P. S. and Sandars, J. (2020). A vision of the use of technology in medical education after the COVID-19 pandemic. *MedEdPublish*, **9**. https://doi.org/10.15694/mep.2020.000049.1.

Hew, K. F. and Lo, K. C. (2018). Flipped classroom improves student learning in health professions education: A meta-analysis. *BMC Medical Education*, **18**: 38. https://doi.org/10.1186/s12909-018-1144-z

Hwang, G. J., Lai, C. L., and Wang, S. Y. (2015). Seamless flipped learning: A mobile technology enhanced flipped classroom with effective learning strategies. *Journal of Computers in Education*, **2**, 449–73.

Isaias, P. (2018). Flipping your classroom: A methodology for successful flipped classrooms. 15th *International Conference on Cognition and Exploratory Learning in Digital Age* (CELDA 2018) ISBN: 978–989–8533–81–4.

Iwai, Y. (2020). 'Online learning during the COVID-19 pandemic: What do we gain and what do we lose when classrooms go virtual?' *Scientific American*. Published 13 March 2020. Available at: https://blogs.scientificamerican.com/observations/online-learning-during-the-covid-19-pandemic/ (accessed 24 March 2020).

Jensen, J., Holt, E. A., Sowards, J. B., Ogden, T. H., and West, R. E. (2018). Investigating strategies for pre-class content learning in a flipped classroom. *Journal of Science Education and Technology*, **27**: 523–35.

Karanicolas, S., Loveys, B., Riggs, K., McGrice, H., Snelling, C., Winning, T. and Kemp, A. (2016). The Rise of the Flip. Successfully engaging students in pre-class activities through the use of technology and a flipped classroom design schema. In S. Barker, S. Dawson, A. Pardo, and C. Colvin (Eds.), *Show Me The Learning* (pp. 312–17). Proceedings ASCILITE 2016, Adelaide.

Khan Academy (2004). What is the History of Khan Academy? Available at: https://support.khanacademy.org/hc/en-us/articles/202483180-What-is-the-history-of-Khan-Academy-.

Khanova, J., Roth, M, T., Rodgers, J, E., McLaughlin, J, E. (2015). Student experiences across multiple flipped courses in a single curriculum. *Medical Education*, **49** (10): 1038–48.

Kim, M. K., Kim, S. M., Khera, O., et al. (2014). The experience of three flipped classrooms in an urban university: An exploration of design principles. *Internet and Higher Education*, 22: 37–50.

Låg, T. and Sæle, R. G. (2019). Does the flipped classroom improve student learning and satisfaction? A systematic review and meta-analysis. *AERA Open*, July–September 5 (3): 1–17.

Lage, M. J., Platt, G. J., and Treglia, M. (2000). Inverting the classroom: A gateway to creating an inclusive learning environment. *The Journal of Economic Education*, 31, 30–43.

Lam, P., Lau, C. K. M., and Chan, C. H. (2019). Collective wisdom of flipped classrooms in Hong Kong higher education: Preparing for potential challenges. The Chinese University of Hong Kong, Hong Kong. *International Conference Educational Technologies 2019*. ISBN: 978-989-8533-83-8.

Lawson, A. P., Davis, C. R., and Son, J. Y. (2019). Not all flipped classes are the same: Using learning science to design flipped classrooms. *Journal of the Scholarship of Teaching and Learning*, 19 (5): 77–104.

Logan, B. (2015). Deep exploration of the flipped classroom before implementing. *Journal of Instructional Pedagogies*, 16.

Loveys, B., Riggs, K., McGrice, H., et al. (2016). *The Rise of the Flip: Successfully Engaging Students in Pre-Class Activities Through the Use of Technology and a Flipped Classroom Design Template*. ASCILITE.

Martin, F., Wang, C., and Sadaf, A. (2018). Student perception of helpfulness of facilitation strategies that enhance instructor presence, connectedness, engagement and learning in online courses. *The Internet and Higher Education*, 37 (2018): 52–65.

Mason, G. S., Shuman, T. R., and Cook, K. E. (2013). Comparing the effectiveness of an inverted classroom to a traditional classroom in an upper-division engineering course. *IEEE Transactions on Education*, 56 (4): 430–5.

McLaughlin, J. E., Roth, M. T., Glatt, D. M., et al. (2014). The flipped classroom: A course redesign to foster learning and engagement in a health professions school. *Acad Med*, 89 (2): 236–43. https://doi.org/10.1097/ACM .0000000000000086. PMID: 24270916.

Miles, C. A. and Foggett, K. (2016). Supporting our students to achieve academic success in the unfamiliar world of flipped and blended classrooms. *Journal of University Teaching & Learning Practice*, 13 (4). Available at: http://ro.uow.edu.au/jutlp/vol13/iss4/2.

Roehl, A., Reddy, S. L., and Gaylajett, S. (2013). The flipped classroom: An opportunity to engage millennial students through active learning strategies. *Journal of Family and Consumer Sciences*, 105 (2): 44–9.

Sams, A. and Bergmann, J. (2013). Flip your students' learning. *Educational Leadership*, 7, 16–20.

Sandrone, S, Berthaud, J, V., Carlson, C., et al. (2020). Active Learning in Psychiatry Education: Current Practices and Future Perspectives. *Frontiers Psychiatry*, 11: 211.

Sezer, B. and Abay, E. (2019). Looking at the impact of the flipped classroom model in medical education. *Scandinavian Journal of Educational Research*, 63:6, 853–68.

Shah, R. and Barkas, L. A. (2018). Analysing the impact of e-learning technology on students' engagement, attendance and performance. *Research in Learning Technology*, 26 (2070). ISSN 2156-7069.

Sharma, N., Lau, C. S., Doherty, I., and Harbutt, D. (2015). How we flipped the medical classroom. National University Hospital, Singapore, The University of Hong Kong, Hong Kong. *Medical Teacher*, 37: 327–30.

Uzir, N. A., Gašević, D., Matcha, W., Jovanović, J., and Pardo, A. (2019). Analytics of time management strategies in a flipped classroom. *Journal of Computer Assisted Learning*, 2020:36; 70–88.

Young, S. and Nichols, H. (2017). A reflexive evaluation of technology-enhanced learning. School of Social Sciences, Leeds Beckett University, Leeds, UK. *Research in Learning Technology*, 25, 2017.

Use of Technology and Social Media

Dr Derek K. Tracy, Dr Patricia Vinchenzo, and Nikki Nabavi

Introduction

Technology and social media have changed psychiatry as much as they have other branches of healthcare. Indeed, we are still learning how to optimise these, and the new risks they carry. This can be a challenge, and one where students may know more than their lecturers. The rapid pace of change always carries the danger of a chapter such as this quickly becoming outdated, but some of the key issues are likely to remain for the foreseeable future, even if individual platforms and applications become redundant, and new ones emerge.

Technology and Psychiatry

Electronic Patient Records to Digital Psychiatry

Electronic patient records (EPRs) have primarily been used as digital versions of old-fashioned 'paper notes', but, properly harnessed, EPRs offer far greater potential to harvest larger data sets and provide better individualised care. At the time of writing, the Royal College of Psychiatrists is updating its core curriculum (RCPsych, 2020a), including a planned new section on digital competencies. This was in recognition that students were taught clinical aspects of mental health, but not how we might utilise technology in their assessment, measurement, and treatment (Dave et al., 2021). Whilst the outcomes of the review were not finalised, the lead author of this chapter was a member of this subgroup, and several key future learning needs on digital literacy were identified:

- Critical appraisal of evidence through digital tools
- Literacy about mental health applications (apps) and 'wearables', including mechanisms of action and side- or adverse effects
- Managing digitally enabled remote consultations, cognisant on emergent challenges to privacy, recording, and safeguarding
- Using EPRs and data science to evaluate clinical records, understand service and individual needs, and change care plans and service provision
- Understanding and managing mental health 'dashboards' and outcome data

Apps and Wearables

The Topol Review (Topol, 2019) provided an overview of and a perspective on preparing the healthcare workforce to deliver a 'digital future'. Addressing this from a mental health perspective, Foley and Woollard (2019) identified key technologies that they argue will significantly impact the mental health workforce in the coming decade. These largely align with the aforementioned proposed RCPsych digital competencies, additionally noting the key role smartphones will play. Such technologies are only emerging at the present time, but are likely to play an important role for the future mental health workforce – and other healthcare – and there should be an open inquiry and detailed discussions with students as to the new technologies' possible risks in a mental health setting. Shah and Berry (2020) discussed and cautioned about the significant rise in venture capital investment in mental health 'digital' to the year 2020, and prospective challenges this may present for us all: they contrast healthcare's dictum of *primum non nocere* ('first, do no harm') with Silicon Valley's 'move fast and break things'.

Conferencing

An outcome of the 2020 coronavirus pandemic was a rapid move to online teaching and conferencing, and at this time it seems likely that the near future will embrace a hybrid model of events retaining a virtual/online component. This opens up novel opportunities, including much easier engagement of a wide range of external speakers and attendees, and pooling work and resources with other, potentially geographically distant, universities and organisations. Live communication between organisers is necessary during a conference, not least as they may be physically separate from each other: this can be through the hosting platform or parallel ones such as Slack. There are indeed excellent opportunities for students to lead such work themselves. We have had very positive experiences of undertaking this (Nabavi et al., 2021), with benefits including:

- Far less time and cost expenses for potential speakers
- Easier access for a wide range of students, including national and international collaboration
- Reduced costs/overheads, which can translate to cheaper tickets/attendance
- Novel functionality such as breakout rooms, different Q&A formats, recording of talks, and enhanced data collection

Social Media and Psychiatry

Blogs

Blogs – a truncation of 'weblog' – have become increasing popular as informal (though styles vary) discussions on topics. At the time of writing, the 'Mental Elf' website (www.nationalelfservice.net) is perhaps the most influential in UK psychiatry, though some universities are housing student work on their own webpages, or on internal servers. At the lead author's primary academic institution (King's College London), Masters' students write blogs as part of their formal assessment, in conjunction with a second piece that involves more traditional evaluation and (systematic or non-systematic) review of a scientific area. We have found that this allows the testing of quite distinct skills: whilst a 'standard' review is good at establishing students' ability to analyse statistical and methodological approaches and assimilate and write up data, blogs focus more on the clear presentation of scientific findings to a lay, but interested, audience. This latter skill is one that will be required by all clinicians throughout their careers as they describe evidence to their patients, whereas the former may be more niche for those in academic careers. If blogs are part of a formal marking process, however, it is crucial to establish any differential marking criteria (e.g. emphasising the use of clear, non-medical language) with students in advance.

Any actual online publication of blogs, whether via the university or in liaison with the Mental Elf website or others hosts, is usually seen as a highly attractive addition to students' CVs. Whilst not 'peer reviewed' in a traditional sense, they are increasingly recognised as demonstrating effort, achievement, and communication skills.

Twitter and Other Platforms

Currently, Twitter is perhaps the dominant social media application in UK psychiatry. It is a commonly used communication tool for individuals, organisations, scientific journals, and learned bodies such as Royal Colleges (Harrison et al., 2019). For lecturers and teaching departments this can be a useful way to communicate with past, current, and prospective students (for psychiatry rotations or for choosing a medical school). For any account representing an institution, permission may be required to use any official logo or branding, and we recommend some form of standard operating procedure on how – and by whom – any such account can be used.

As well as a communication forum for students, Twitter can be a mechanism to find and highlight new research and clinical developments in mental health, advertise local events and achievements, hear from opinion leaders, and engage in conversations with others with whom one might otherwise ordinarily not cross paths. Psychiatry and psychiatrists have been commendable as a profession in engaging trainees and others, deconstructing the common medical hierarchy. Social media can be a considerable source of factually incorrect information and disinformation (Grimes et al., 2020); greater critical thought will need to be given to what is found via social media in comparison to more traditional sources such as peer-reviewed journals.

Other social media platforms are available, contemporaneously including Facebook, Instagram, LinkedIn, and, most recently, TikTok. Each has varying strengths, depending upon what one is trying to achieve. In our experience, Facebook can be helpful as a local forum for a PsychSoc (see section on 'PsychSocs, Virtual Journal Clubs, and Student-to-Student Engagement') or university department to 'host events' and act as a news feed; it encourages individuals to click 'going' to or 'interested' in events, which in turn helps generate excitement, promotes appearance of the event on others' news feeds, and so forth. It can also be a means of advertising positions and opportunities to students, and to publish local articles and magazines. Instagram can also be a good platform for engaging in topical conversations around mental health, stigma, and well-being, with the ability to post videos and photos; currently, however, its use is typically greater amongst student populations and it is less commonly used professionally by qualified practitioners (albeit with some notable exceptions). LinkedIn is most commonly used by individuals to showcase their professional achievements, and is perhaps more common in the commercial sector than in healthcare or academia, but departments may find this another mechanism to advertise their work to a different audience. TikTok has been used in healthcare to convey brief healthcare video messages, including to the public. It is newer than the other formats, and its utility is less clear at this time. The broader point is, perhaps, to recognise that every platform will carry unique opportunities, and good educators will work with their students in determining the value and roles of each.

PsychSocs, Virtual Journal Clubs, and Student-to-Student Engagement

Most universities will have a psychiatry society or 'PsychSoc'. The Royal College of Psychiatrists supports these practically through modest financing and by providing access to a national bank of speakers, thus also offering a platform for networking with other PsychSocs (RCPsych, 2020b). In recent times, PsychSocs have proved to be both influential and dynamic (Pandian et al., 2020) in helping encourage and support students, destigmatise psychiatry and mental illness, and innovate in broadening the syllabus beyond traditional core teaching. This has included attracting national and international speakers and linking up with other medical specialties (e.g. psychological aspects of oncology). PsychSocs by their nature will contain committed and enthusiastic individuals, many of whom will be more familiar with the use of technology and who can engage other students in ways traditional lecturers cannot.

A recent development, partially led by PsychSocs, has been the running of online journal clubs. This offers many of the advantages noted in the section on conferences, though with far less work required. It can also serve to stimulate presenting students to allow and encourage wider access to the journal club. Innovative examples have included inviting an author of the paper to engage – something usually quite difficult in all but the most uncommon of face-to-face circumstances – and having other experts (including patients) and policy makers involved. *The British Journal of Psychiatry* has started running a national virtual journal club with interested PsychSocs and teaching departments: such involvement, and that of other organisations, can also be stimulating and exciting for students, and can tap into a larger pool of potential additional speakers (BJPsych, 2020).

Some caution and thought, however, will be required for events broadcast outside of the classroom: consideration will need to be given to the possibility that what is said may be recorded: patient confidentiality is paramount, and language and tonality must be particularly respectful. It is also likely that some students may be reluctant and nervous at such prospects, and wider engagement should really be optional.

Well-Being and Privacy on Social Media

New challenges are emerging as a result of the use of social media, and guidelines have been issued by the General Medical Council (GMC, 2013), the British Medical Association (BMA, 2018), and the Royal College of Psychiatrists (RCPsych, 2020c). The main principles of these are summarised in Table 5.3.1. These are worth discussing with students, as well as with any staff new to the tools. A key challenge is whether to maintain discrete accounts for personal and professional use. Whilst we are all entitled to a personal life, it is a reality that medical students' and doctors' online behaviours is liable to be held up to public scrutiny, and our profiles may be searched by our patients and employers. There are already examples of medical students and doctors being referred to the GMC because of things they have posted, and unfortunate – but real – examples of how social media profiles might be adversely viewed by hiring clinical or academic institutions with regard to ascertaining doctors' 'professionalism' (Tracy et al., 2020).

Conversely, there are challenges to the well-being of students and professionals online. It has become increasingly well documented that many individuals have been subjected to harassment and bullying online: those posting from professional perspectives can face additional risks of this kind, and these should be discussed with students. Furthermore, the 'democratisation' of social media means that people can convey medical disinformation,

Table 5.3.1 A summation of key points from GMC, BMA, and RCPsych guidelines on doctors' use of social media

- Treat patients and colleagues fairly and with respect, maintaining public trust in the profession
- Remember that any postings may be seen by current or future patients, universities, and employers, and that some might intentionally search your online history
- Maintain patient confidentiality at all times
- Respect appropriate professional boundaries with current or potential patients
- If you identify yourself as a doctor in publicly accessible media, you should also identify yourself by name
- Consider having a separate private/anonymised account where you can share personal interests and activities with friends and family; you might wish to tighten the security settings and limit who can view this
- Signposting to information sources is usually not problematic, but there are significant risks in giving personalised health advice, and this should be avoided
- In general, try avoid posting online when angry or upset, or after consuming alcohol
- Remember that defamation law applies online; avoid unsubstantiated comments
- Do not forget that individual postings may carry unintended implications for one's university, hospital, etc.
- Be transparent about any conflicts of interest that you might have

some potentially harmful ('anti-vaccination' and 'anti-medication' postings being notable). Professionals and students may feel a need to try to engage with such postings, but this can be challenging (Grimes et al., 2020); students should consider if they are best placed to redress this, and any risks of so engaging.

On the one hand, we must all accept that not everyone has had a good experience with mental health services or professionals, and expressions of diverse opinions and perspectives on issues such as psychotropic medication are valid even if contrary to the evidence base. These should generally be accepted in good faith, even if not endorsed or agreed with, and uncivil arguments avoided (Rimmer, 2020). Despite the perceived 'democratisation' of voices on social media, many service users may feel that medical students' and professionals' opinions will be treated more seriously. On the other hand, 'trolling' and abuse of anyone should not be tolerated, even taking into account that in some instances hostile posting may be driven by individuals' mental ill-health. Most social media platforms have mechanisms for complaining about such postings, but students should be encouraged to seek any required mentoring support. Not responding to aggressive messaging and taking breaks from social media are key skills for professionals to develop.

Conclusion

Technology and social media are making enormous changes to medical education, teaching, and practice. They bring substantial and as yet not fully understood opportunities in terms of diversifying and democratising conversations and information, and in breaking down many traditional barriers of geography and cost. However, they raise two major forms of challenge: the first is that their rapid change can make it difficult to keep up with what is topical and in contemporaneous use – here the solution can be mutual learning from doctor–student conversations. The second is the challenge to professionalism, both in terms of what medical students and doctors post online and the implications of this, and he risks of various forms of online harassment and bullying. Sensible, pragmatic education will recognise these balances and work with them, rather than ignoring their use.

References

BJPSYCH. (2020). *Improving access to research* [Online]. Cambridge University Press. Available: www.cambridge.org/core/journals/the-british-journal-of-psychiatry/information/improving-access-to-research (accessed 20 October 2020).

BMA (2018). *Social media, ethics, and professionalism*. London: British Medical Association.

Dave, S., Abraham, S., Ramkisson, R., et al. (2021). Digital psychiatry and COVID19: The big bang effect for the NHS? *BJPsych Bull*, 45 (5): 259–63. https://doi.org/10.1192/bjb.2020.114. PMID: 33081867; PMCID: PMC7844168.

Foley, T. and Woollard, J. (2019). *The digital future of mental healthcare and its workforce*. London: Higher Education England.

GMC. (2013). *Doctors' use of social media*. London: General Medical Council.

Grimes, D. R., Brennan, L. J., and O'Connor, R. (2020). Establishing a taxonomy of potential hazards associated with communicating medical science in the age of disinformation. *BMJ Open*, 10, e035626.

Harrison, J. R., Hayes, J. F., Woollard, J., and Tracy, D. K. (2019). #BJPsych and social media – likes, followers and leading? *Br J Psychiatry*, 214, 245–7.

Nabavi, N., Vinchenzo, P., and Tracy, D. K. (2021). Learning in the time of Covid: How to organise a virtual medical conference. *BMJ Student*, m4942.

Pandian, H., Mohamedali, Z., Chapman, et al. (2020). Psych Socs: Student-led psychiatry societies, an untapped resource for recruitment and reducing stigma. *BJPsych Bull*, 44, 91–95.

RCPSYCH. (2020a). Curricula and guidance. Royal College of Psychiatrists. Available: www.rcpsych.ac.uk/training/curricula-and-guidance (accessed 20 October 2020).

RCPSYCH. (2020b). PsychSocs. Royal College of Psychiatrists. Available: www.rcpsych.ac.uk/become-a-psychiatrist/med-students/psychsocs (accessed 20 October 2020).

RCPSYCH (2020c). *Social Media Staff and Members Policy*. London: Royal College of Psychiatrists.

Rimmer, A. (2020). How do I deal with criticism online? *BMJ*, 371, m3978.

Shah, R. N. and Berry, O. O. (2020). The rise of venture capital investing in mental health. *JAMA Psychiatry*. https://doi.org/10.1001/jamapsychiatry.2020.2847.

Topol, E. (2019). *The Topol Review. Preparing the healthcare workforce to deliver the digital future*. London: Higher Education England.

Tracy, D. K., Joyce, D. W., Albertson, D., and Shergill, S. S. (2020). Kaleidoscope. *Br J Psychiatry*, 217, 593–4.

Quality in Medical Education

Dr Genevieve Holt and Dr Miranda Kronfli

Introduction: What is 'Quality' and Why is it Important?

Involvement in education happens at all stages of a doctor's career and can take many forms. For most, it includes informal roles such as ad hoc teaching in clinical settings or completing assessments for junior colleagues in the workplace. Other clinical educators take on more formal roles, for example as undergraduate tutor, medical school year-lead or campus subdean. No matter the formality of the role, or the regularity of the teaching, it is vital to consider the quality of the educational input being provided; understanding basic principles of how learning occurs, and keeping abreast of advances in education research are fundamental to this. Ensuring a robust, pedagogically sound design is however, not enough. It is essential to anticipate, when planning the design and delivery of your course, how you will know if it is any good. How will you define 'good', anyway? You might consider whether your course is fit for purpose. You might ask yourself if it justifies the resources spent on it, in terms of curriculum weighting, educator time, and budget. Or you might check that it fits with the goals of those who are involved in the programme, both directly and more broadly.

Defining quality is a challenge (Harvey and Green, 1993), but there are some commonly held values which help to structure quality practices, such as: 'added value' (Vroeijenstijn, 1995); fitness for purpose; meeting or exceeding internal and external standards, monitoring, and consistency (Harvey and Green, 1993). Considering quality as a way of looking at both the processes and the outcomes of teaching and assessment (Harvey and Green, 1993) offers a helpful way to consider what practical steps might be needed. There are significant parallels in how standards are set, maintained, and improved for both clinical work and medical education, although the frameworks used in different settings are often circumscribed according to the primary occupation of individual practitioners. Those whose roles are primarily patient-facing or concerned with delivery of clinical services will be involved in local clinical governance activity, including Quality Improvement (QI), while medical educators employed by higher education institutions (HEI) may be familiar with Quality Assurance (QA) or Quality Assurance and Enhancement (QAE) processes.

In this and the following chapter, we aim to equip those involved in the design and delivery of learning and teaching interventions, whatever their level or type of involvement in undergraduate education, with an understanding of some of the basic principles and practices of quality in medical education. We will share some tools for your practice to help you to frame useful questions, and to help in your pursuit of quality in your teaching, learning, and assessment endeavours in undergraduate education and in disseminating your work.

How Can We Frame Quality Endeavours?

Defining 'Quality'

An important first step is to consider who defines what may be counted as 'quality'. There is no universal definition of 'quality' in medical education. This is partly because different people or groups apply different meanings of the term, depending on their interest in the intervention – or, to put it another way, 'Quality is in the eye of the beholder' (Vroeijenstijn, 1995). The General Medical Council (GMC) reminds us that in all our governance endeavours, the safety and positive experience of patients is the main goal. Those involved in medical education have a wider 'social accountability', a responsibility to patients and society, which means they must work with relevant groups and organisations, and fulfil relevant requirements as part of their accreditation processes (Kenwright and Wilkinson, 2018). Professional regulators such as the GMC are key stakeholders in the quality of undergraduate medical education, and safeguard this using dedicated monitoring processes. Students also have their own understanding of what good 'quality' education means, and taking this into account is strongly advocated in the literature relating to 'Students as Partners' in education (Healey et al., 2014). There are thus many perspectives from which 'quality' might be defined, and the need to consider these means that it is important to involve a variety of different 'stakeholders' when carrying out quality endeavours (Vroeijenstijn, 1995).

Secondly, there are many different elements of quality which can be selectively incorporated into any QI or QA endeavour. The different meanings of quality held by different parties refer to 'different things with the same label' (Harvey and Green, 1993, p. 3). This means that when setting out your goals it is important to describe clearly what is meant by quality, and what this means for how you carry out your quality endeavour. As well as fitness for purpose or value for money (Harvey and Green, 1993), quality has been considered as signifying diverse concepts: for example, authentic partnership with students (Healey et al., 2014), proactive attention to the interests of stakeholders (Vroeijenstijn, 1995), ongoing improvement of processes (Vroeijenstijn, 1995), and quality as culture or attitude (Cardoso et al., 2016; Dolmans et al., 2011).

Perceptions of quality change over time, with new definitions emerging and old ones becoming obsolete as wider social and cultural values change. An increasing recognition of the need for equity of access to medical school has resulted in Widening Participation initiatives. These are designed, among other goals, to develop a diverse workforce and promote opportunities to those from under-represented groups (Rees and Woolf, 2020), based on characteristics such as socio-economic status, disability, and ethnicity (BMA, 2020; Selecting for Excellence Executive Group, 2014).

As we can see, the practice of quality is applied across different domains of education, including the learning environment, learning outcomes, learning methods, and assessment (Kenwright and Wilkinson, 2018), and is undertaken in a variety of ways (as described later in the chapter).

What are the Different Types of Quality-Related Practice?

Through their clinical work, healthcare professionals are frequently exposed to quality processes, with a focus on ensuring patient safety, QA, and QI, to maintain and improve the quality of services (GMC, 2013). QI places emphasis on a structured method, applied by providers and stakeholders, in order to sustainably transform system performance (Health Foundation, 2013). These facets of clinical governance are coordinated at an organisational level, with communities of clinical staff engaged in ways which correspond to their clinical and managerial roles. Those working within the frame of an HEI should familiarise themselves with institutional and regulatory QA processes that their educational provision is subject to.

Healthcare professionals who are involved in teaching often undertake their work as educators somewhat – or even entirely – removed from the organisational structures that are responsible for the undergraduate psychiatry curriculum and accountable for education quality. These individuals may not have insight into the relevance of quality processes or the expertise to carry them out. Ad hoc teaching can occur in clinical settings and may be undertaken by medical, nursing or allied professional staff in workplace settings where students attend placements. They may provide teaching opportunistically, or arrange structured education sessions with varying degrees of formality, without ever being aware of the wider context in which psychiatry learning has been planned. It is important that all those involved in teaching, learning, and assessment gain the skills needed to attend to the quality of their teaching – not just those who are accountable to external stakeholders in formal QA processes. It is therefore necessary to set out in detail the main approaches, and offer some specific guidance regarding how to implement them.

Historically, several practices have informed the way. The most common quality-related practices which medical educators currently undertake to ensure quality of their educational interventions are QI and QA, with Quality Enhancement emerging in higher education as a more recent term (Cardoso et al., 2019). The distinction between these terms in practice is discussed in more detail later and will be relevant to different educators in different ways. Depending on the setting, certain practices are more common than others, as each process has different characteristics which make it suited to the function it serves.

The process that many healthcare professionals will be familiar with is QI. This concept evolved from industry, where standardisation of components on an assembly line was crucial to the quality of the end product. Statistical analysis of data is now routinely applied in manufacturing in order to drive improvement, and more recently these techniques have been adapted for use to improve quality in healthcare settings. QI in healthcare is now used to describe a continuous process of identifying and addressing opportunities for improvement.

QA has been defined as 'a process of measuring attributes of a course or programme against internal or external standards' (Kenwright and Wilkinson, 2018, p. 103). It is thus a formal process which allows higher education departments to monitor the quality of their programmes using a variety of process and outcome measures, and assure stakeholders of this quality. These stakeholders can be internal stakeholders such as the university or student bodies, or external stakeholders such as regulatory bodies (the GMC is an important stakeholder in QA of undergraduate programmes) and the Quality Assurance Agency (QAA).

QA processes are sometimes thought of as summative, providing an opportunity for course leads to communicate to those to whom they are accountable that a course meets expected standards. QI can be considered as a more formative, ongoing process, designed to explore in depth the factors which are influencing success or failure (Kenwright and Wilkinson, 2018). In practical terms, however, the distinction is not as clear, with many aspects of QA (such as dialogue with students and iterative programme evaluation) being exploratory and developmental, and not confined to the end of a programme.

Contemporary Issues in Educational Quality

A 'Critical' Approach to Quality

As important as it is to make sure that we have ways of ensuring our educational interventions meet the objectives that we, and others, have for them, it can also be helpful to step back and question the QA or QI process itself – for example, asking how is this process working?', 'who is responsible for this process?', or 'what is this process achieving?' Questioning the value and approach to quality in this way, rather than automatically taking the approach at face value, is known as taking a 'critical' approach to quality (Bleakley et al., 2013). A critical approach can be helpful in several ways. Considering which definition of quality is being used, or from whose perspective 'quality' has been defined, can help us to understand, for example, to what end a QA or QI process is being employed. If we note that in a particular project quality seems to be defined as, to take one example, efficiency, we might understand that our evaluation (and, in turn, perhaps also the design and delivery of the educational intervention), is being driven from a 'managerial' viewpoint. We might notice that viewpoints such as the 'profession-alism' viewpoint, or the pedagogic, scientific, or ethical viewpoints (Bleakley et al., 2013), are less influential in the process. This 'noticing' might help us to remember to also prioritise other drivers that are important to us, such as pedagogic robustness or important social values.

Quality Culture

Dolmans et al. (2011) recognise that despite a robust evaluation approach, even one that is thoroughly executed, something additional is needed for improvement to occur and to be sustained. For quality endeavours to result in tangible improvement, cultural change is needed. This relies on an ability to influence the attitudes, values, and beliefs of those involved in programme design and delivery. This includes, at times, the learners themselves. Many learners are used to a model wherein the educator's word is final, and may have strong expectations of how they might be involved in the quality process. Several elements can contribute to a 'quality culture': for example, a sense of ownership of the process among those involved (Bleakley et al., 2013), alignment with institutional strategy (Griffin and Cook, 2009), good working relationships (EUA, 2006), supportive leadership (Kenwright and Wilkinson, 2018), and a culture of scholarship in teaching and learning (Lovato and Peterson, 2018).

References

Academy of Medical Educators. (2015). About AoME. Available at: www .medicaleducators.org/About-AoME (accessed 5 July 2020).

Association for Medical Education in Europe. (2020). About AMEE. Available at: https:// amee.org/what-is-amee (accessed 5 July 2020).

Association of University Teachers of Psychiatry. (2020). What is the AUTP.

Available at: https://www.autp.org/home (accessed 4 April 2022).

Biggs, J. B. (2011). *Teaching for quality learning at university: What the student does.* McGraw-Hill Education.

Bleakley, A., Browne, J., and Ellis, K. (2013). Quality in medical education. In T. Swanwick, K. Forrest, and B. C. O' Brien (eds), *Understanding Medical Education: Evidence, Theory, and Practice* (pp. 47–59),

2nd ed. Wiley Blackwell. https://doi.org/10.1002/9781118472361.ch4.

British Medical Association (2020). Widening Participation in Medicine. Available at: https://www.bma.org.uk/advice-and-support/studying-medicine/becoming-a-doctor/widening-participation-in-medicine#:~:text=Widening%20participation%20(WP)%20is%20a,from%20low%20socio%2Deconomic%20groups (accessed 1 November 2020).

Cardoso, S., Rosa, M. J., and Stensaker, B. (2016). Why quality in higher education institutions is not achieved? The view of academics. *Assessment and Evaluation in Higher Education*, **41**: 950–65.

Cardoso, S., Rosa, M. J., Videira, P., and Amaral, A. (2019). Internal quality assurance: A new culture or added bureaucracy? *Assessment & Evaluation in Higher Education*, **44** (2): 249–62.

Crampton, P., Mehdizadeh, L., Page, M., Knight, L., and Griffin, A. (2019). Realist evaluation of UK medical education quality assurance. *BMJ Open*, **9** (12): e033614.

Creswell, J. W., 2014. *A concise introduction to mixed methods research*. SAGE publications.

Dolmans, D. H. J. M., Stalmeijer, R., Van Berkel, H., and Wolfhagen, I. H. A. P. (2011). Quality assurance of teaching and learning: Enhancing the quality culture. In T. Dornan, K. V. Mann, A. J. Scherpbier, and J. A. Spencer (eds.), *Medical Education: Theory and Practice* (pp. 257–64). Edinburgh: Churchill Livingston, Elsevier Ltd.

European University Association. (2006). Quality Culture in European Universities: A bottom-up approach: Report on the three rounds of the Quality Culture project 2002–2006. Available at: https://eua.eu/resources/publications/656:quality-culture-in-european-universities-a-bottom-up-approach.html (accessed 4 April 2022).

Frye, A. W. and Hemmer, P. A. (2012). Program evaluation models and related theories: AMEE guide no. 67. *Medical Teacher*, **34** (5): e288–e299.

General Medical Council. (2013). Good Medical Practice. Available at: www.gmc-uk.org/ethical-guidance/ethical-guidance-for-doctors/good-medical-practice (accessed 4 April 2022).

General Medical Council. (2015). Promoting excellence: standards for medical education and training. Available at: www.gmc-uk.org/-/media/documents/Promoting_excellence___guide_for_stakeholders.pdf_63751869.pdf (accessed 4 April 2022).

Greene, L. and Prostko, C. R. (2010). Educational Needs Assessment, Activity Development, and Outcomes Assessment at PRIME: Applications of Established Conceptual Frameworks and Principles of Adult Learning. Available at: https://primece.com/science-of-cme/adult-learning-principles/ (accessed 5 July 2020).

Griffin, A. and Cook, V. (2009). Acting on evaluation: Twelve tips from a national conference on student evaluations. *Medical Teacher*, **31** (2): 101–4.

Haji, F., Morin, M. P., and Parker, K. (2013). Rethinking programme evaluation in health professions education: Beyond 'did it work?' *Medical Education*, **47** (4): 342–51.

Harvey, L. and Green, D. (1993). Defining quality. *Assessment & Evaluation in Higher Education*, **18** (1): 9–34.

Healey, M., Flint, A., and Harrington, K. 2014. Engagement through partnership: Students as partners in learning and teaching in higher education. www.heacademy.ac.uk/sites/default/files/resources/engagement_through_partnership.pdf (accessed 4 April 2022).

Health Foundation. (2013). Quality Improvement Made Simple: What Everyone Should Know About Quality Improvement. Available at: www.health.org.uk/sites/default/files/QualityImprovementMadeSimple.pdf (accessed 24th October 2020).

Holt, G., Ryland, H., and Shah, A. (2017). Quality improvement for psychiatrists. *British Journal of Psychiatry Advances*, **23**, 206–14.

Jorm, C. and Roberts, C. (2018). Using complexity theory to guide medical school evaluations. *Academic Medicine*, **93** (3): 399–405.

Kenwright, D. N. and Wilkinson, T. (2018). Quality in medical education. In T. Swanwick, K. Forrest, and B. C. O' Brien (eds), *Understanding Medical Education: Evidence, Theory, and Practice* (pp. 101–10), 2nd ed. Wiley Blackwell.

Kirkpatrick, D. (1967). Evaluation of training. In R. L. Craig and L. R. Bittel, eds. *Training and Development Handbook*. New York: McGraw-Hill, 87–112.

Kolb, D. A. (1984). *Experiential learning: Experience as the Source of Learning and Development* (Vol. I). Englewood Cliffs, NJ: Prentice-Hall.

Kolb, D. A. (2015). *Experiential Learning: Experience as the Source of Learning and Development*. 2nd ed. Upper Saddle River, NJ: Pearson Education.

Lovato, C. and Peterson, L. (2018). Programme evaluation. In T. Swanwick, K. Forrest, and B. C. O' Brien (eds), *Understanding Medical Education: Evidence, Theory, and Practice* (pp. 443), 2nd ed. Wiley Blackwell. https://doi.org/10.1002/9781119373780.ch30.

Mayhew, E. (2019). Hearing everyone in the feedback loop: Using the new discussion platform, Unitu, to enhance the staff and student dialogue. *European Political Science*, 18 (4): 714–28.

Miller, G. E. (1990). The assessment of clinical skills/competence/performance. *Academic Medicine*, 65 (9): S63–7.

Rees, E. and Woolf, K. (2020). Selection in context: The importance of clarity, transparency and evidence in achieving widening participation goals. *Medical Education*, 54 (1): 8–10.

Selecting for Excellence Executive Group. (2014). Selecting for excellence final report. Available at: www.medschools.ac.uk/media/1203/selecting-for-excellence-final-report.pdf (accessed 01 November 2020).

Vroeijenstijn, A. I. (1995). Quality assurance in medical education. *Academic Medicine*, 70 (7 Suppl): S59–67.

Wong, G., Greenhalgh, T., Westhorp, G., and Pawson, R. (2011). Realist methods in medical education research: What are they and what can they contribute? *Medical Education* 46 (1): 89–96.

Quality in Practice

Dr Miranda Kronfli and Dr Genevieve Holt

In the previous chapter we discussed some of the principles and meanings of 'Quality' in Clinical Education and saw how important it is to consider the quality of any educational intervention, whichever part of the process you are involved in: design, implementation, or delivery. In this chapter, we set out specific elements of the processes of Quality Improvement (QI), and Quality Assurance (QA), with the aim of providing some practical ways for you to consider quality in your own clinical education role.

Quality Improvement: Learning for Improvement in Clinical Practice and Education

In our everyday lives we are always learning; we harness the feedback generated by an experience and use it as we move on to the next experience. This innate tendency to continuously learn and improve is formalised by QI, which provides a structure to introduce changes and learn about their impact on a system. It demands a rigorous, systematic approach to complex systems – those with multiple, interrelated components – to understand change and drive improvements.

Tools to undertake iterative learning experiments for the purposes of improving quality have been developed but, depending on the field in which they are employed, clinicians and educators might well describe similar concepts using different language and models. The two cycles outlined here relate to how learning occurs, and both have their origins in science and technology.

Kolb's Experiential Learning Cycle

Those with an interest in education are likely to have encountered David Kolb's experiential learning cycle, a theory published in 1984 that recognises the role of experience in learning. Kolb's theory of learning draws on intellectual origins, including the work of Kurt Lewin, a social psychologist who borrowed concepts from electrical engineering and applied them to behavioural sciences. Although Kolb's cycle is often applied to the process of learning by students, it can also be used to understand how a teacher continuously learns and develops in the role of medical educator.

This four-stage cycle documents the process of learning, dividing it into the following components: experiencing (concrete experience), reflecting (reflective observation), thinking (abstract conceptualisation), and acting (active experimentation).

Plan-Do-Study-Act Cycle

Clinicians with exposure to QI will have come across a cycle known as Plan-Do-Study-Act (PDSA; see Figure 6.2.1); this iterative four-step learning loop facilitates testing of a hypothesis that an improvement team hopes will result in improvement. PDSA is based on scientific methodology and developed from the manufacturing industries, popularised by William Deming following World War II.

PDSA encourages systematic preparation for a change (plan) that is then carried out (do), reflected upon using relevant data from the test of change (study), and then proceeds with further tests of change (act). It facilitates learning by the team who 'continuously build knowledge using an evidence base that is accumulated through their own practice' (Holt, Ryland, and Shah, 2017, p. 208) when the cycle is used iteratively.

Figure 6.2.1 PDSA cycle

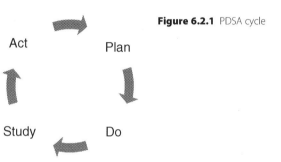

Act

Plan

Study

Do

Several similarities can be noted between the two models set out here; each features an experience from which learning will be derived, explicitly requiring data about the experience to be interrogated and reflected upon as the basis for future development. These data, in the case of individual educators, medical education departments, and education institutions, will frequently comprise feedback about teaching that has been delivered as well as measures such as student (or teacher) attendance and student performance in assessments.

Improving the Quality of Teaching

With these well-established models in mind, it is possible for individual educators to structure improvements to their own teaching offerings, whatever the scale of educational activity, and to capture the steps for achieving this. Application of these models to teaching can also be undertaken with the support of peer educators or in a professional peer group, with a view to enhancing the process of reflection and engaging in a richer dialogue. Innovations to teaching, if documented so they align with the PDSA cycle, have the potential to be framed as QI initiatives which will create additional opportunities for dissemination of knowledge about psychiatry teaching and how it can be optimised in the specific settings where it occurs.

Quality Assurance: Ensuring Outcomes Meet Expectations

Quality Assurance Processes

QA can be broadly described as a process of identifying standards, setting goals (for evaluation, implementation of change, and dissemination of findings), collecting and analysing evaluation data, investigating unanticipated findings, planning and implementing change, and disseminating the findings to relevant stakeholders. It is applied to all processes of medical undergraduate education, from admissions to course implementation (Kenwright and Wilkinson, 2018). The evaluation goals which inform the design of the QA process depend on which qualities need to be demonstrated, and the goals of those involved, such as learners, commissioners, regulators, and patient groups, for example. As well as allowing those who lead an education programme to demonstrate the quality of the programme to such stakeholders, information gathered can be used to help educators to develop the programme, as part of a process of iterative evaluation.

Internal and External Standards

Depending on the level of educational intervention being considered, the process of identifying standards must consider internal factors, including intended learning outcomes of the intervention, aims of the programme lead or educator, institutional QA requirements, and the expressed needs of learners both past and present. External standards must also be adhered to: for example, the expectations of regulators such as the Quality Assurance Agency and the General Medical Council, and education commissioners such as Health Education England (HEE).

QA is an important aspect of any medical undergraduate curriculum. The GMC (General Medical Council) set standards for medical education and training with five discrete themes: Learning Environment and Culture, Educational Governance and Leadership, Supporting Learners, Supporting Educators, and Developing and Implementing Curricula and Assessments (GMC, 2015). These standards include require-ments which must be met by organisations and which are regularly assessed by the GMC through performance monitoring and visits to institutions. Such external stakeholder QA standards and agendas have been shown to be of value to providers of undergraduate medical education (Crampton et al., 2019), for example providing powerful opportunities for leverage for those seeking to make changes within their own organisations.

Setting Goals

The above-noted standards, in combination with the evaluator's considerations of priority and feasibility, will inform the goals of the QA process. Goals can be flexible, for example if they are influenced by unexpected findings or newly arising feasibility constraints. Consultation should take place with stakeholders to ensure that quality is assessed in line with their expectations, which may need to be balanced with those of faculty or learners (Vroeijenstijn, 1995).

Evaluation of teaching interventions should be planned during the design phase of teaching. Setting clear goals by asking questions such as 'What will I want to demonstrate I've achieved?' can help guide a more considered and robust design. These goals will then inform identification and design of appropriate tools for data collection and analysis, and for reporting and dissemination.

Programme Evaluation

Evaluation is an important step in the QA process, allowing insight into the process and/or outcomes of an education intervention, enabling communication with stakeholders regarding the efficacy of a programme, and assisting in the planning of iterative design and development (Lovato and Peterson, 2018).

A robust evaluation will be focussed, successful in meeting its goals, useful, and sufficiently well designed and executed to justify its findings. A clear evaluation strategy, set out at the start, clearly describing what success will look like and setting clear and achievable goals, is vital, and can also be important way to signal to potential stakeholders (such as funders, commissioners, or potential collaborators) that an education project is likely to be successful.

A common evaluation approach is to assess whether a programme achieves previously identified outcomes. Quasi-experimental designs are commonly employed for this purpose. Kirkpatrick's (1967) hierarchy for evaluating training interventions has been widely adopted as a way of identifying educational outcomes against which to evaluate and has been adapted for use in healthcare settings (Greene and Prostko, 2010). Other theoretical models useful for conceptualising educational outcomes for evaluation include Miller's framework for assessment of clinical skills, competence, and performance (Miller, 1990), and Biggs' theory of Constructive Alignment (Biggs and Tang, 2015).

Given the value of identifying the complex mechanisms that influence the success or otherwise of an intervention, there is a case for moving beyond the 'outcome' model, to evaluating *how* an intervention works (Haji, Morin and Parker, 2013). This takes into account the complexity of the intervention and its context (Frye and Hemmer, 2012). Approaches such as Realist Evaluation (Wong et al., 2011) or complexity theory (Jorm and Roberts, 2018) are increasingly used for process evaluation (Crampton et al., 2019; Frye and Hemmer, 2012).

Collecting and Analysing Data

The choice of method for collecting and analysing evaluation data depends on the goals of the QA process. Although often done at the end of an educational intervention to inform summative communication of the quality of the programme, it can be valuable to conduct evaluation during the course of a programme – for example, to inform iterative programme development, or to reassure stakeholders that the programme is progressing appropriately. Some approaches to data collection are set out in Table 6.2.1 below.

Dialogic Feedback

Allowing more informal opportunities for feedback can be a valuable way to create genuine dialogue with students (Griffin and Cook, 2009), compared to more traditional methods such as confining feedback to formal processes like end-of-programme evaluation forms. This allows students to draw on their own conceptions of quality when feeding back, rather than being constrained by definitions of quality represented in questionnaire constructs, which are defined by members of faculty. Ways to collect feedback more informally include generic feedback email addresses (Griffin and Cook, 2009), dedicated discussion forums within online modules, ad hoc questions from tutors during live teaching (remote and in-person), and electronic student voice platforms such as Unitu[TM] (Mayhew, 2019). These platforms allow students to 'upvote' and 'downvote' peers' comments, supporting a degree of quantification of findings and allowing educators to prioritise programme developments.

Table 6.2.1 Data collection methods

Data Collection Methods	Potential Advantages	Examples
Quantitative approaches	Valuable to demonstrate accountability to external or internal stakeholders If a research design is required (e.g. if dissemination plans include publication in a peer-reviewed journal), using a published, validated questionnaire can help to support robust quantitative findings	Questionnaires, employing rating scales (e.g. Likert scales) Electronic voting apps such as Mentimeter Polls within videoconferencing platforms such as Blackboard Collaborate (specifically designed for use in educational settings) or Zoom
Qualitative approaches	Allow the collection of detailed information about how and why a programme is working (or not working) Inform iterative development of an educational intervention Allow unanticipated findings to be captured	Free-text questionnaire questions are often used to collect qualitative data from a large number of participants Focus groups allow the evaluator to explore specific concepts in greater depth, workshop potential changes for implementation, or gather more information about issues identified on questionnaires Individual or group interviews allow more detailed, in-depth exploration of specific issues
Mixed methods approaches	Can employ both qualitative and quantitative approaches Commonly used to demonstrate impact and illuminate barriers and facilitators to its achievement 'Exploratory' models allow evaluators to identify phenomena during an initial qualitative phrase, and then measure them by subsequently collecting quantitative data 'Explanatory' models allow educators to use free-text questions to explain unexpected quantitative results (Cresswell, 2014)	Inviting learners to give feedback using Post-it notes offers a potentially anonymised and immediate way to gather feedback from face-to-face sessions, which can be analysed qualitatively or quantitatively Voting apps such as Mentimeter allow the same to be done for live sessions conducted remotely using video conferencing platforms

Once collected, acting on student feedback, and telling students how this has been done, is not only an effective way to create dialogue with students, but is also an important part of 'closing the loop' in the quality cycle (Griffin and Cook, 2009).

Collaborative discussion with students (e.g. at Staff–Student Consultative Committees) regarding how to respond to evaluation findings allows educators to ensure that any change that forms part of the QA process is relevant to students' own experience. Any suggestions from students should be balanced against the expertise of the faculty and professional services staff, and students should understand that, for this reason, not all suggestions will be implemented. It is important that other considerations relevant to a student partnership approach be made – for example, ensuring students are compensated for their time (Griffin and Cook, 2009), perhaps by applying for funding from local student partnership initiatives.

Quality Assurance and Enhancement in Different Settings

Educational interventions designed to support the learning of medical students occur in a variety of settings, with degrees of formality varying from formal delivery of their undergraduate programme in the HEI setting, to informal learning opportunities in the clinical workplace. The way in which the attendance to the quality of learning in these settings might be conceptualised varies according to the type of educational intervention being offered; the professional sphere of the organisation, team, or individual offering it; and the theoretical school of thought which influences that field. Appendix 6.2.1 includes examples that illustrate, for a clinical educator involved in design or delivery of educational interventions, how provision of quality might be considered.

Disseminating Good Practice: Submitting Your Write Up

Research in medical education is conducted from a different viewpoint to traditional clinical research, in that it draws on a variety different of academic disciplines and deals with social phenomena (such as people and their behaviours) rather than biomedical phenomena (like the action of different medications in the body). For many clinical educators, resolving this tension to the point where they feel comfortable seeking publication of education work can be a difficult journey. Starting with a literature review is crucial, providing an opportunity to consolidate your own understanding of the topic – including education theory relevant to your intervention – and to help you, as an author, understand what novel learning you will add to the body of research. A key foundation for successfully progressing research and evaluation projects to publication is ensuring, from the outset, that you have a robust design framework that adheres to the methodological principles of the relevant field – for example, QI or evaluation. Increasing familiarity with QI methodology amongst clinicians provides a useful stepping-stone for those who are interested in presenting or publishing in medical education spheres, as QI acknowledges the importance of a specific environment in which changes are tested and places considerable value on documenting and finding ways to share qualitative experience, in common with medical education research.

There are several organisations specialising in disseminating learning about medical education, and those involved in undergraduate psychiatry teaching who wish to share their experiences and learning in this area might find these useful starting points (see Table 6.2.2).

Table 6.2.2 Potential avenues for dissemination

Organisation	Brief summary
The Association of University Teachers of Psychiatry (AUTP)	UK-based organisation that seeks to improve standards in psychiatry teaching at both undergraduate and postgraduate levels. An annual conference provides opportunities to share ideas and learning, showcasing education projects and approaches in psychiatric medical education. Membership is open to those multidisciplinary professionals involved in teaching psychiatry to medical learners or students in related professions (AUTP, 2019).
The Academy of Medical Educators (AoME)	A UK-based organisation, AoME aims to provide leadership, promote standards, and support those involved in medical education. This remit of this multiprofessional group includes all stages of education and continuing professional development for medical, veterinary, and dental learners. It supports educators to demonstrate expertise and achievements in medical education through accreditation as a medical teacher, to an agreed national standard (AoME, 2015).
The Association for Medical Education in Europe (AMEE)	This is an international organisation that promotes excellence in education in the health professions across undergraduate, postgraduate, and continuing education. It holds annual conferences and provides a platform for disseminating work in the field of medical education via several publications (AMEE, 2020).
The Association for the Study of Medical Education (ASME)	A UK-based organisation which aims to support research-informed best practice in medical education. They have dedicated career groups for students (JASME) and trainees (TASME) to support those developing their education practice with opportunities for publication and presentation.

Further Reading

Programme Evaluation

Frye, A. W. and Hemmer, P. A. (2012). Program evaluation models and related theories: AMEE guide no. 67. *Medical Teacher*, **34** (5): e288–e299.

Methods of Data Collection and Analysis

Lovato, C. and Peterson, L., 2018. Programme evaluation. In T. Swanwick, K. Forrest, and B. C. O' Brien (eds), *Understanding*

Medical Education: Evidence, Theory, and Practice (pp. 443), 2nd ed. Wiley Blackwell.

Contemporary Issues in Quality

Bleakley, A., Browne, J., and Ellis, K. (2013). Quality in medical education. In T. Swanwick, K. Forrest, and B. C. O' Brien (eds), *Understanding Medical Education: Evidence, Theory, and Practice* (pp. 47–59), 2nd ed. Wiley Blackwell. https://doi.org/10.1002/9781118472361.ch4.

References

Academy of Medical Educators. (2015). About AoME. Available at: https://www.medicaleducators.org/About-AoME (accessed 5 July 2020).

Association for Medical Education in Europe. (2020). About AMEE. Available at: https://amee.org/what-is-amee (accessed 5 July 2020).

Association of University Teachers of Psychiatry. (2020). What is the AUTP. Available at: www.autp.org/home (accessed 4 April 2022).

Biggs, J. B. (2011). *Teaching for quality learning at university: What the student does*. McGraw-Hill Education.

Biggs, J. and Tang, C. (2015). Constructive alignment: An outcomes-based approach to teaching anatomy. In L. K. Chan and W. Pawlina (eds.), *Teaching Anatomy* (pp. 31–8). Cham: Springer.

Bleakley, A., Browne, J., and Ellis, K. (2013). Quality in medical education. In T. Swanwick, K. Forrest, and B. C. O' Brien (eds), *Understanding Medical Education: Evidence, Theory, and Practice* (pp. 47–59), 2nd ed. Wiley Blackwell. https://doi.org/10.1002/9781118472361.ch4.

British Medical Association (2020). Widening Participation in Medicine. Available at: https://www.bma.org.uk/advice-and-support/studying-medicine/becoming-a-doctor/widening-participation-in-medicine#:~:text=Widening%20participation%20(WP)%20is%20a,from%20low%20socio%2Deconomic%20groups (accessed 1 November 2020).

Cardoso, S., Rosa, M. J., Videira, P., and Amaral, A. (2019). Internal quality assurance: A new culture or added bureaucracy? *Assessment & Evaluation in Higher Education*, **44** (2): 249–62.

Crampton, P., Mehdizadeh, L., Page, M., Knight, L., and Griffin, A. (2019). Realist evaluation of UK medical education quality assurance. *BMJ Open*, **9** (12): e033614.

Creswell, J. W. (2014). *A concise introduction to mixed methods research*. SAGE Publications.

European University Association. (2006). Quality Culture in European Universities: A bottom-up approach: Report on the three rounds of the Quality Culture project 2002–2006. https://eua.eu/resources/publications/656:quality-culture-in-european-universities-a-bottom-up-approach.html (accessed 4 April 2022).

Frye, A. W. and Hemmer, P. A. (2012). Program evaluation models and related theories: AMEE guide no. 67. *Medical Teacher*, **34** (5): e288–e299.

General Medical Council. (2013). Good Medical Practice. Available at: www.gmc-uk.org/ethical-guidance/ethical-guidance-for-doctors/good-medical-practice (accessed 4 April 2022).

General Medical Council. (2015). Promoting excellence: standards for medical education and training. Available at: www.gmc-uk.org/-/media/documents/Promoting_excellence_guide_for_stakeholders.pdf_63751869.pdf (accessed 4 April 2022).

Greene, L. and Prostko, C. R. (2010). Educational Needs Assessment, Activity Development, and Outcomes Assessment at PRIME: Applications of Established Conceptual Frameworks and Principles of Adult Learning. Available at: https://primece.com/science-of-cme/adult-learning-principles/ (accessed 5 July 2020).

Griffin, A. and Cook, V. (2009). Acting on evaluation: Twelve tips from a national conference on student evaluations. *Medical Teacher*, **31** (2): 101–4.

Haji, F., Morin, M. P., and Parker, K. (2013). Rethinking programme evaluation in health professions education:Beyond 'did it work?' *Medical Education*, **47** (4): 342–51.

Harrington, K., Flint, A., and Healey, M. (2014). Engagement through partnership: Students as partners in learning and teaching in higher education. www.heacademy.ac.uk/sites/default/files/resources/engagement_through_partnership.pdf (accessed 4 April 2022).

Harvey, L. and Green, D. (1993). Defining quality. *Assessment & Evaluation in Higher Education*, **18** (1): 9–34.

Health Foundation. (2013). Quality Improvement Made Simple: What Everyone Should Know About Quality Improvement. Available at:

www.health.org.uk/sites/default/files/Quality ImprovementMadeSimple.pdf (accessed 24th October 2020).

Holt, G., Ryland, H., and Shah, A. (2017). Quality improvement for psychiatrists. *British Journal of Psychiatry Advances*, **23**, 206–14.

Jorm, C. and Roberts, C. (2018). Using complexity theory to guide medical school evaluations. *Academic Medicine*, **93** (3): 399–405.

Kenwright, D. N. and Wilkinson, T. (2018). Quality in medical education. In T. Swanwick, K. Forrest, and B. C. O' Brien (eds), *Understanding Medical Education: Evidence, Theory, and Practice* (pp. 101–10), 2nd ed. Wiley Blackwell.

Kirkpatrick, D. (1967). Evaluation of training. In: R. L. Craig and L. R. Bittel, eds. *Training and Development Handbook*. New York: McGraw-Hill, 87–112.

Lovato, C. and Peterson, L. (2018). Programme evaluation. In T. Swanwick, K. Forrest, and B. C. O' Brien (eds), *Understanding Medical Education: Evidence, Theory, and Practice* (pp. 443), 2nd ed. Wiley Blackwell. https://doi.org/10.1002/9781119373780.ch30.

Kolb, D. A. (1984). *Experiential learning: Experience as the Source of Learning and Development* (Vol. **1**). Englewood Cliffs, NJ: Prentice-Hall.

Kolb, D. A. (2015). *Experiential Learning: Experience as the Source of Learning and Development*. 2nd ed. Upper Saddle River, NJ Pearson Education.

Mayhew, E. (2019). Hearing everyone in the feedback loop: Using the new discussion platform, Unitu, to enhance the staff and student dialogue. *European Political Science*, **18** (4): 714–28.

Miller, G. E. (1990). The assessment of clinical skills/competence/performance. *Academic Medicine*, **65** (9): S63–7.

Rees, E. and Woolf, K. (2020). Selection in context: The importance of clarity, transparency and evidence in achieving widening participation goals. *Medical Education*, **54** (1): 8–10.

Selecting for Excellence Executive Group. (2014) Selecting for excellence final report. Available at: www.medschools.ac.uk/media/1203/selecting-for-excellence-final-report.pdf (accessed 1 November 2020).

Vroeijenstijn, A. I. (1995). Quality assurance in medical education. *Academic Medicine*, **70** (7 Suppl): S59–67.

Wong, G., Greenhalgh, T., Westhorp, G., and Pawson, R. (2011). Realist methods in medical education research: What are they and what can they contribute? *Medical Education*, **46** (1): 89–96.

Appendix
Practice Examples

• Evaluating Professional Development Teaching in a Medical School

Asif is a clinical teaching fellow at a medical school. He has been asked by the Year 1 Lead to evaluate the Professional Development module for first year undergraduates. The Year Lead is keen to better understand students' experience, as there have been some low scores recently and they are aware there is a routine internal inspection planned in eighteen months' time.

Having taught on the programme for two years, Asif is aware that Student Evaluation Questionnaires (SEQs) are sent out at the end of the module, but the response rate is poor. He feels that a different approach to evaluation might work better. Asif discusses a potential redesign with the Year 1 Lead, who suggests he makes an Evaluation Plan that both takes into account the evaluation requirements of the university and his own expertise as programme tutor. After consulting the relevant section of the University Academic Regulations, Asif understands that the SEQs are compulsory, that they include some mandatory questions, and that the results are regularly disseminated to the faculty as part of the faculty QA process. He also finds out that the university has a new Education Strategy which places a new emphasis on working in partnership with students to evaluate programmes, and that funds have been set aside for new student partnership evaluation projects. Asif decides to apply for funding to support the development of his evaluation strategy. During the process of applying, Asif learns that applicants are asked to demonstrate how students' own conceptions of quality are incorporated into the evaluation of programmes and also to indicate how students will be informed about the impact of their feedback. Asif also has had several ideas for how to improve the programme during his two years as tutor, based on his conversations with students, and is therefore keen to ensure that tutors can contribute to the evaluation.

Asif makes an evaluation plan which sets out two clear goals: to gain insight into students' experience on the module, and to identify some clear goals for development of the module based on students' experience. He decides that to justify any changes to the year lead he would like to collect some quantitative data. He is also aware that he will need to collect some qualitative data from students, to understand students' own conceptions of 'quality', if his application for funding for a student partnership project is to be seriously considered. Asif therefore includes three data collection tools in his evaluation plan: A student evaluation questionnaire with quantitative Likert-style questions (including the mandatory questions set by the university); free-text questions oriented at understanding students' own goals for the programme and their conceptions of how the programme succeeded or failed in meeting those goals; and separate focus groups with students and faculty to allow exploration of any negative feedback (quantitative or qualitative). Asif hopes that his funding application will be accepted to allow him sufficient resource to facilitate, transcribe, and analyse the focus group data. However, in case the application is not accepted, he makes a plan to use existing institutional structures to allow dialogue with students and staff. For example, he plans to workshop ideas with student representatives at the termly Staff–Student Consultative Committee. He plans to use monthly tutor meetings to allow student reps' ideas to be discussed with tutors and the programme lead in order to identify suitabl development goals for the programme and ensure that his second evaluation goal i addressed. Asif takes his plan to the Year Lead, who endorses it and also suggests that h ensures that the discussions with faculty include the programme administrator. They sugges that he includes a dissemination goal to create a bulletin for the student magazine, te communicate how students' input has informed development of the programme.

Reflection

What are the set requirements of the institution in relation to the evaluation you are carrying out?

What will you want your evaluation to demonstrate you've achieved?

How will you make sure students feel that the process is relevant to them, and how will you communicate your findings and their impact to students?

Will you want to publish your evaluation? If so, how will you demonstrate the following?.

- That your intervention robustly designed and is seated in the relevant education theory
- That your intervention was successful and adds something new that other similar interventions don't already do
- That your evaluation strategy reflects what you are trying to achieve and is designee appropriately to evidence this
- That your write up will offer something that others who read it might find useful
- That your evaluation methods were robust enough to allow you to justify the conclusion you draw; for example, is your sample size big enough, did you pilot your questionnaire what method of data analysis did you use, were any focus groups conducted in a way which minimised bias?

Have you thought about the above questions early enough in the process for it to be meaningful?

2   Psychiatry Placement

Heather is a psychiatry core trainee who is interested in medical education. She provide weekly teaching sessions for groups of five undergraduate medical students who are or placement in the Trust. The placements last four weeks, following which a new group o students rotate into psychiatry. She works in a Trust with a QI programme and has learn about PDSAs which are being used for QI in clinical settings; Heather thinks it will be usefu to use what she has learnt about PDSAs in her teaching activity.

Initially, Heather planned sessions based on her own expertise, gained whilst working or an inpatient ward for people with severe dementia. The students, however, also brough questions related to their own experiences of clinical psychiatry – for example, observation: from acute psychiatry wards for working-age adults and things they had seen wher shadowing junior doctors on-call.

Heather develops a teaching timetable; she obtains a copy of the undergraduate psych-iatry curriculum and aligned her teaching with the undergraduate learning objectives. She captures reflections about her teaching in a logbook and obtains anonymous feedback from the students after each session, having adapted a feedback form used by the local medical education team. Heather is able to collect both qualitative (free-text comments) and quantitative (rating scales) information; every time she delivers a session, Heather uses these data to inform her lesson plan for her next teaching slot.

Heather wonders if she could use her teaching experience by way of a quality improvement project, so contacts one of the QI leads in her area. Their discussion brings Heather to the realisation that she can continue to improve the quality of her teaching using PDSA cycles as she has been doing, without the need for QI methodology. This will be a more efficient use of her time, as QI would require a team of stakeholders meeting regularly and statistical analysis of data without adding sufficient value to her endeavours to justify the investment. However, the QI lead encourages her to write up her work and seek publication, as she has kept careful documentation of her approach and other educators might find it useful to understand how she has adapted tools used in QI for educational purposes. Heather obtains the support of the undergraduate psychiatry tutor for the medical school and they produce a paper together, presenting their work at a regional education conference.

Reflection

What does 'quality' mean in your work as an educator, and who has decided this?

What sources of information do you already have access to that can tell you something about the quality of your work in education?

Would it be beneficial to access additional sources of information or consider other measures of quality?

Gathering Feedback

Dr Laura Sharp, Dr Dimitar Karadzhov, and Dr Helena Paterson

As illustrated in the previous chapter, it is valuable to embed a cyclical model of curriculum enhancement focused on incorporating feedback on the student experience, intended learning outcomes, and professional skills acquisition into the teaching provision. When implemented systematically, thoughtfully, and collaboratively as part of this quality improvement cycle, student feedback becomes a powerful mechanism for improving the learning experience (Fullana et al., 2016; Biwer et al., 2020; Deeley et al., 2019). Gathering systematic student feedback on various aspects of the teaching provision is instrumental in increasing the constructive alignment of the curriculum. Constructive alignment refers to the degree of synergy between intended learning outcomes, assessment structures, and students' learning practices and outcomes (Biggs, 1996).

Collating feedback which explores the alignment of course resources with professional standards provides an opportunity to strategically establish ways of enhancing good practice and identify areas that require development. Student feedback should be collected at multiple points of course delivery, particularly at the course design stage, during the course, and at course completion (see Figure 6.3.1). The feedback gathered during these stages serves interrelated but distinct functions in terms of quality enhancement. For instance, during the course, feedback can be collected regularly – both formally and informally (e.g. via discussion forums or during lectures) – to identify practical issues that could be addressed swiftly, as well as to encourage deeper student reflection. Upon course completion, educators can follow up on pertinent issues raised by the students and engage in a more comprehensive examination of how this feedback could be incorporated into the future teaching provision. In all cases, educators can use feedback to open dialogues with students in order to clarify student expectations and identify steps towards meeting these.

Lived Experience

Gordon Johnston

When people with lived experience, or any external contributors, are involved in the delivery or facilitation of teaching sessions, it is valuable to seek immediate student feedback on their satisfaction with, and perceived impact of, those sessions. It is also good practice to seek feedback from the contributors themselves in relation to their experience of the planning and delivery of the teaching. This can lead to positive reinforcement when things have gone well and to constructive ideas for improvement when necessary.

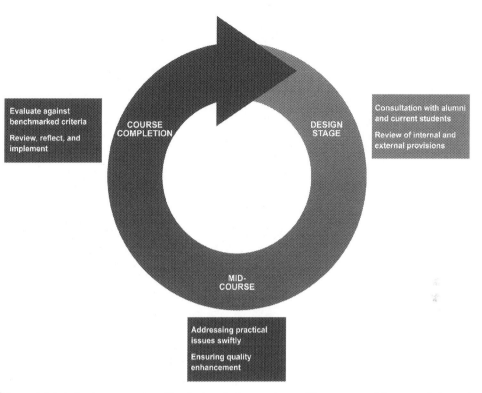

Figure 6.3.1 A visual representation of feedback-gathering practices at different stages of the course design and delivery.

Transparency, collaboration, and continuity are among the overarching principles governing effective collection and use of feedback (Deeley et al., 2019). These can be advanced by clearly communicating with students how their feedback has been interpreted and what its role as a mechanism for quality enhancement is. The processes of student evaluations, staff–student liaison, and emergent actions can be shared with future cohorts to allow students to see how the student voice has influenced the teaching provision in concrete ways. Ideally, students should be positioned as partners within the collective endeavour to design rigorous, effective, and useful teaching.

There is a diversity of data-gathering methods available for eliciting students' evaluations of, and experience with, course delivery (Sharp et al., 2018) Available at: https://sites .kowsarpub.com/jme/articles/105640.html. For example, traditional review techniques such as surveys could be pragmatically complemented by participatory methods such as collaborative workshops (Sharp et al., 2018; Cohen et al., 2013; Cowan and George, 2013). Adopting a multifaceted approach to feedback allows educators to gain insights into the student experience, while also encouraging students to build self-efficacy through guided reflection. Some of the advantages and limitations of different types of feedback-gathering approaches are compiled in Table 6.3.1.

There is a wide range of topics, experiences, and processes about which to seek feedback. Different approaches to collecting this information can be employed depending on a range

Table 6.3.1 Advantages and limitations of different types of feedback-gathering techniques

	Advantages	Limitations
Surveys	Can be administered to large numbers of students Quick and easy to administer Anonymous Suitable for obtaining a 'snapshot' of student perceptions and experiences in real time Can be utilised for efficient quality monitoring and control Can inform deeper discussion in workshops	Survey items may be ambiguous or misleading Driven largely by educators' agenda and priorities Responses lack context and may be difficult to interpret Poor response rates may limit their usefulness
Collaborative workshops and focus groups	Can elicit rich, contextualised responses Learner-centred and solution-oriented (Cohen et al., 2013) Promote equality and democracy (Cohen et al., 2013; Fullana et al., 2016) Can probe effectively into the process of student learning, into students' emotions, motivation, and moments of challenge or perplexity (Fullana et al., 2016; Bush and Bissell, 2008)	Time-consuming to plan and execute Typically conducted with small, unrepresentative samples May elicit large amounts of qualitative data, making them impractical to employ regularly with large student cohorts Less amenable to standardisation and comparison Lack anonymity, which may hinder recruitment

of factors, including time-frames, resources, and class size. For instance, feedback gathered on an assignment can serve to elicit information on students' newly acquired knowledge, their perceived pedagogic value of the assignment, and preparation approaches, as well as encourage reflection on the processes and outcomes of learning (Castle et al., 2014). These can focus on the learning, teaching, and course organisation or, more generally, on the professional value of the skills being targeted. Course evaluations could target a range of aspects of the curriculum and the student experience (see Table 6.3.2). To maximise the usefulness and authenticity of the feedback, evaluation questions should target both students' positive experiences *and* any challenges faced during the course. Illustrative examples of the various approaches to feedback gathering are available in the Appendix. These include generative prompts for student discussions applied in our own practice of teaching psychology, global mental health, and genetic counselling (Sharp et al., 2018; Cowan and George, 2013).

Table 6.3.3 presents several overarching principles for gathering quality feedback informed by the broader pedagogic literature and applied in our own practice.

Negative student feedback is not uncommon, which tends to trigger a range of affective reactions in educators (Simpson and Siguaw, 2000; Moore and Kuol, 2005). Students may give negative feedback for various reasons. For instance, their learning experience might have diverged considerably from what they expected or were promised by course leads. Such negative feedback could be indicative of the existence of a 'hidden curriculum', which is likely to impede optimal learning and teaching practices (Blasco, 2012). The 'hidden

Table 6.3.2 Examples of feedback questions about different aspects of the teaching provision

Curriculum components and aspects of the student experience	Exemplary evaluation questions
Engagement with the virtual learning environment (VLE)	Please explain how you approached engaging with the online learning materials over time
Optimal workload and timetabling	To what extent did the timetable work efficiently for you?
Constructive alignment between curriculum, intended learning outcomes (ILOs), assessments, and/or graduate attributes	To what extent did the curriculum support the attainment of the course ILOs?
Usefulness of different resource types, learning modalities, and learning software (e.g. podcasts, lectures, blended learning, forums, quizzes)	What is your preferred learning resource format from the course, and why?
Responsiveness to student needs and skills development	Were you offered adequate opportunities to develop the skills to effectively engage with the learning materials at the start of the programme?
Assessments – their format, timing, alignment with ILOs, usefulness for developing transferable skills, and other attributes	Can you think of examples of how the assessments in this course are supporting your professional skills development?

Table 6.3.3 Principles for gathering quality feedback

1. Utilise various sources and techniques, such as self-report measures and performance-type measures (Biwer et al., 2020). This helps corroborate findings and minimise both student and educator biases.
2. Ensure inclusivity and accessibility by using jargon-free and neutral language, as well as by having a diverse representation of respondents (Locke et al., 2013).
3. Boost the number of responses by sending frequent reminders, offering incentives and demonstrating respect for students' opinions (Nulty, 2008).
4. Incentives should be used with caution as their misuse may lead to coercion (Nulty, 2008).
5. Assess the pros and cons of different survey formats. While paper-based surveys may yield greater response rates, online surveys better protect anonymity (Nulty, 2008).
6. Be transparent: tell students how their feedback is going to be used and provide evidence of how past feedback has informed the teaching provision (Cohen et al., 2013).
7. Minimise the student burden of participation in course evaluations by carefully planning the timing, volume, and length of evaluation surveys.
8. Secure informed consent and protect students' confidentiality (Cohen et al., 2013).
9. Be mindful that student feedback may not always reflect the quality of teaching (Carpenter et al., 2020). Students may not have an insight into the multitude of useful curriculum components or their intended effects on learning and career progression (Carpenter et al., 2020; Stark and Freishtat, 2014; Kornell, 2020).

curriculum' refers to the mismatch between stated curriculum goals and principles (i.e. how students *are expected* to learn) and the realities of student learning (i.e. how they *actually* learn), which has been linked to poorer learning and satisfaction outcomes (Sambell and McDowell, 1998; Blasco, 2012). Routine evaluations of student attitudes, satisfaction, and learning practices are instrumental in bringing the 'hidden curriculum' to light.

It is important that educators have a clear mechanism for responding to feedback, including feedback that is negative or appears harsh or personally critical. Educators should first focus on processing any negative feelings before enacting appropriate, thoughtful, and constructive responses (Simpson and Siguaw, 2000; Moore and Kuol, 2005).

Student evaluations of teaching remain the cornerstone of quality assurance, accountability, and curricular innovation in higher education. The effectiveness of feedback gathering is shaped by a multitude of factors, of which educators' best practice knowledge, skills, and aptitudes are fundamental.

References

Biggs, J. B. (1996). Enhancing teaching through constructive alignment. *Higher Education*, **32**: 347–64.

Biwer, F., Oude Egbrink, M. G., Aalten, P., and de Bruin, A. B. (2020). Fostering effective learning strategies in higher education – A mixed-methods study. *Journal of Applied Research in Memory and Cognition*, **9** (2): 186–203.

Blasco, M. (2012). Aligning the hidden curriculum of management education with PRME: An inquiry-based framework. *Journal of Management Education*, **36** (3): 364–88.

Bush, H. and Bissell, V. (2008). The evaluation of an approach to reflective learning in the undergraduate dental curriculum. *European Journal of Dental Education*, **12** (2): 103–10.

Carpenter, S. K., Witherby, A. E., and Tauber, S. K. (2020). On students' (mis) judgments of learning and teaching effectiveness. *Journal of Applied Research in Memory and Cognition*, **9**, 137–51.

Castle, D., Sanci, L., Hamilton, B., and Couper, J. (2014). Teaching psychiatry to undergraduates: Peer-peer learning using a 'GP letter'. *Academic Psychiatry*, **38** (4): 433–7.

Cohen, L., Manion, L., and Morrison, K. (2013). *Research methods in education*. Abingdon: Routledge.

Cowan, J. and George, J. (2013). *A handbook of techniques for formative evaluation: Mapping the students' learning experience*. Abingdon-on-Thames: Routledge.

Deeley, S. J., Fischbacher-Smith, M., Karadzhov, D., and Koristashevskaya, E. (2019). Exploring the 'wicked' problem of student dissatisfaction with assessment and feedback in higher education. *Higher Education Pedagogies*, **4** (1): 385–405.

Fullana, J., Pallisera, M., Colomer, J., et al. (2016). Reflective learning in higher education: A qualitative study on students' perceptions. *Studies in Higher Education*, **41** (6): 1008–22.

Hadwin, A. F., Winne, P. H., Stockley, D. B., et al. (2001). Context moderates students' self-reports about how they study. *Journal of Educational Psychology*, **93** (3): 477.

Kornell, N. (2020). Why and how you should read student evaluations of teaching. *Journal of Applied Research in Memory and Cognition*, **9** (2): 165–9.

Locke, T., Alcorn, N. and O'Neill, J. (2013). Ethical issues in collaborative action research. *Educational Action Research*, **21** (1): 107–23.

Moore, S. and Kuol, N. (2005). Students evaluating teachers: Exploring the importance of faculty reaction to feedback on teaching. *Teaching in Higher Education*, **10** (1): 57–73.

Nulty, D. D. (2008). The adequacy of response rates to online and paper surveys: What can be done? *Assessment and Evaluation in Higher Education*, **33** (3): 301–314.

QAA (2018). UK Quality Code for Higher Education (online). Available at: www.qaa.ac.uk/quality-code

Sambell, K. and McDowell, L. (1998). The construction of the hidden curriculum: Messages and meanings in the assessment of student learning. *Assessment & Evaluation in Higher Education*, **23** (4): 391–402.

Simpson, P. M. and Siguaw, J. A. (2000). Student evaluations of teaching: An exploratory study of the faculty response. *Journal of Marketing Education*, **22** (3): 199–213.

Sharp, L., Karadzhov, D. and Langan Martin, J. (2018). The curious case of blended learning: An evaluation of a curriculum innovation in the global mental health Master's programme. *Journal of Medical Education*, **17** (3): 149–59.

Stark, P. and Freishtat, R. (2014). *An evaluation of course evaluations*. ScienceOpen. Center for Teaching and Learning, University of California, Berkley (online). Available at: www.scienceopen.com/hosted-document?doi=10.14293/S2199-1006.1.SOR-EDU.AOFRQA.v1 (accessed 4 April 2022).

UK Professional Standards Framework. (2011) (online). Available at: www.heacademy.ac.uk/system/files/downloads/UKPSF%20Dimensions%20of%20the%20framework.pdf

Appendix

Minute note	Informal Online or paper Qualitative

Request that students take one minute to provide a written response to a set question. This can provide the educator with insight into student engagement and understanding. This feedback can highlight misunderstandings but also inform appropriate directions for future teaching sessions. Educators may collate the minute note responses and engage them as an opener for their next session. In addition, the opportunity to communicate informally through scraps of paper may open dialogue with students who opt to add additional queries or feedback in their submission.

Take 1 minute to note down the key takeaway messages from this learning session.

Post-It Notes	Informal Paper Qualitative

Provide students with 'post-it' notes and wall space (s) to stick their response to. This approach can be particularly useful for exploring 'strengths and limitations' or 'positives and negatives'. These can help gain a better understanding of student experience and can also inform future quantitative questions in the form of a questionnaire.

What aspects of the learning resources work well? What are the benefits of this approach?

What aspects of the learning resources DO NOT work well? What are the challenges or barriers of engaging with online learning resources?

The Power of Experience	Informal Online or paper Qualitative

Request that students reflect on their knowledge and experience. This can inform future communication by educators. For example, sharing this information with the next cohort of students can demonstrate to them that student input is important and offer them direction with their study plans.

What would I have told my younger self if they were completing this course?
What pearls of wisdom would you pass on to next year's students?

SKS: Stop Keep Start	Informal Paper Qualitative

Request that students respond to these three questions. This can provide a valuable overview of what students consider to be surplus to requirements, what they value, and ideas for future development. These questions can be targeted at course delivery, course content, or programme organisation.

What should I / we STOP?
What should I / we KEEP?
What should I / we START?

In-class or Online Discussions	Informal Online or in-class Observation of responses

Pose a question that encourages students to engage personal observations as well as to explore the literature. This is an informal approach for educators to gather feedback about student comprehension and to identify areas and topics which need further focus. In this exemplar, students were provided with some key learning materials on triggers and sources of trauma and asked to contribute to an online discussion forum.

Reflect on whether chronic life adversity such as community violence is likely to cause similar types of traumatic experiences as acute adversity such as a natural disaster or a life-changing medical diagnosis.

Educators can input into, and direct, the discussion to promote opportunities for a range of key learning topics to be explored. In this exemplar, these may include:
That different types of traumas affect different people in different ways. Therefore, it may not be beneficial to try and generalise the effects that different kinds of trauma have on people.
That acute traumatic events may be more likely to be recognised as being traumatic than certain types of chronic and environmental traumas.
Consideration of the implications of being born into an environment where chronic trauma already exists and growing up and living in this environment (i.e. the cultural norms individuals are exposed to).
Potential benefits of trying to find commonalities in people who have been exposed to the same kind of trauma.

Key Demographic Information	Formal Online or paper Quantitative Questionnaire or workshop
Collate key quantitative responses to allow varying student experiences to be explored by group to identify trends. Potential questions include:	
Please select the most accurate description for you:	UK student EU student International student
Is English your first language?	Yes No (I am a non-native English speaker) Other (please specify)
What is your gender?	Female Male Other (please specify)
Location of study	On campus Online distance learner
Are you studying:	Full-time Part-time

Brief – 4 question CPD feedback	Formal Online or paper Quantitative and qualitative
Engage quantitative and qualitative questions to provide an overview of student experience. In this exemplar a specific student group (General Practitioners – GPs) undertaking Continual Professional Development (CPD) were targeted by a brief questionnaire to determine their perceived value of a learning resource focussing on suicide prevention.	
Have you found this course helpful for your day-to-day work as a GP?	Yes No
Are you more confident in opening conversations with patients about feelings of suicide in your GP clinic?	Yes No
Would you recommend this course to GP colleagues?	Yes No
For your CPD, what is your one key learning point from this course?	

Evaluation: New Formative Assessment	Formal Online or paper Quantitative and qualitative
Conduct a brief survey to evaluate student experiences of a new resource. This exemplar enquired about the utility of a formative assessment, which involved three 'pre-assessment' stepped activities. Educators were interested in students' experiences of the three activities (draft submission, comparison, and reflection) and the impact the activities had on students' approach to assignment completion.	
Do you think the academic value of the formative pre-assessment activities was made clear?	Yes No Could have been clearer
Which of the pre-assessment activities did you submit?	None Step 1 – Draft submission Steps 1 and 2 – Draft submission and comparison All steps (steps 1, 2 and 3) – Draft submission, comparison and reflection
(Filter question determined by response to question above) **What would have increased the likelihood of you engaging with all the pre-assessment activity steps?**	
The pre-assessment activities were accompanied with clear and sufficient instructions.	Strongly agree Agree Neither agree not disagree Disagree Strongly disagree
The pre-assessment activities made me feel more confident about completing the summative assignment.	Strongly agree Agree Neither agree not disagree Disagree Strongly disagree

Collaborative workshop (exploring survey feedback)	Formal Discussion Qualitative

Conduct a workshop to explore the interpretation of feedback from a questionnaire. In this exemplar students completed an end of programme survey considering a range of topics including the learning materials, course organisation, and assessments. It was apparent that the current assessment approach was unsatisfactory for some students and the education team was interested in gaining additional clarification on some of the issues. Some key questionnaire findings were presented to a smaller cohort of students in a workshop environment followed by some discussion questions.

Questionnaire feedback:

Almost a quarter (24%) of the original questionnaire respondents considered the timing between assessment submissions deadlines to be inappropriate. In qualitative responses five students indicated that the assessment timings could be stressful or intense and two indicated that the combination of formative and summative assignments made coursework feel overwhelming. 18% of students identified a specific poster assignment as most difficult to complete whilst a different 18% identified a systematic review as most challenging.

Discussion themes:

Establish what the issues with the submissions were.
Identify which assignments caused challenges, and why.
Establish if the students were aware that all assignment information and deadlines were available at the beginning of each term.
Clarify when students started assignment planning and completion.
Explore why a considerable proportion of the students considered the poster assignment and the systematic review to be most challenging.

The Student in Difficulty

7.1

Dr Angela Cogan

It would be wonderful if medical school was exciting, enjoyable, interesting, and fulfilling for all medical students at all times, however, most students will face periods of adversity during their medical school degree. In most cases this is normal and to be expected; the issue is transient, is solved either via the student's own personal resource, using their natural support systems or with help from a professional, and does not contravene the boundaries of professionalism. However, sometimes the concern runs deeper than this. Medical students are the doctors of the future, in whom patients will one day place their health and their lives (General Medical Council, 2016b). They often feel there are real barriers to asking for help and worry about the consequences should they do so. It is important that they are provided with the necessary support to navigate through these difficulties whilst remediating, growing, and learning from the issues identified, with patient safety central to this ethos.

Medical Students Can Encounter Problems for a Number of Reasons

There is no doubt that medical students can face significant pressure – but why is this? The answer is complex, and is different in every case. Academic pressure starts from day one and the workload can soon build up if students do not keep on top of it. Students may be leaving home for the first time and working out how to look after themselves, trying to find their way around a new city let alone just round the university campus, working out how to keep to a budget, make new friends, and have the challenge of keeping up with a demanding course and learning to study in ways which may be completely new to them.

Medical school is very different from school. Although some are graduates with other degrees, most medical students have to learn to adapt to a changed work and study environment. Ways of learning that worked previously may not prove effective at medical school, and the volume of work may be vastly greater. Students may find it tricky to manage their time. Keeping a healthy work/life balance is important, but often students let their outside interests slip in trying keep up with the volume of work or fail to prioritise measures to maintain their well-being and physical and mental health.

The medical degree course itself is distinctive from most other university courses in that there is a difference in the expected standard of behaviour compared to students studying other subjects (General Medical Council, 2016b). Some students can struggle with this expectation, which in turn leads to increased pressure and strain. Social media is an increasingly common context for lapses in professionalism. Education on the responsible use of social media and associated risk awareness must be embedded within medical school curricula (O'Regan et al., 2018).

Medical students can build up significant amounts of debt during their years at medical school. Financial worries can impact negatively on students' well-being and performance (Ross et al., 2006), and some may be concerned that they are not able to pay for travel to their placement or afford the costs of daily living such as rent and food. Medical students often have part-time jobs in addition to their full-time studies. This can lead to insufficient time for studies or to working late at night with associated tiredness during the day. Whilst helpful in paying off debt and building up finances, working during holiday periods can mean that medical students fail to have a break that leaves them refreshed for the oncoming session.

Medical students have to cope with their own personal life events whilst being exposed to instances of human suffering within their curriculum that are likely to have an emotional impact. It is important that we provide students with safe ways to share and reflect on these difficult experiences and role model this in practice. Medical students may have relatives who see them as 'the medical member of the family' and may need support in learning to set boundaries in this area.

Medical students have higher rates of depression, suicidal ideation, other mental illness, and burnout than the general population (Schwenk et al., 2010). Their worries concerning stigma they may face from their medical school or future profession are well documented (Schwenk et al., 2010), and it is important that as a profession and as individuals we are able both to challenge this view and to support students with mental illness. The jointly developed GMC document entitled 'Supporting medical students with mental health conditions' (GMC, 2015) is a helpful resource for medical students and those involved in teaching. Students may present with physical ill health. In addition, their own concerns about their health may be brought into focus when faced with similar illnesses in others.

Medical students come from a diversity of backgrounds and life circumstances. Overseas medical students may have particular support needs due to a lack of familiarity with their new home and work environment (General Medical Council, 2016b). Students can experience significant stress due to micro-aggressions or perceptions of 'other' within the medical school environment – for example, due to factors such as race, gender, or economic status – and this experience is not acceptable. Diversity in the student population should be celebrated, and medical schools have a responsibility to provide support tailored to their diversity of needs. Medical schools may have extra provision for students who are part of a widening participation programme or may have clinical placements who are 'carer friendly' for students with caring responsibilities. Students who are carers may have significant environmental stressors and responsibilities and can feel torn between these and the need to focus on their studies.

Relationship issues are often to the fore. Family members sometimes fail to understand or lack sympathy for the demands of the medical school degree. Friction with family members, partners, peers, and with or between other flatmates can place the student under significant strain and is often not easily ameliorated. Students worry about their peers and their duty of care to each other. They will come to us with worries regarding friends and classmates. This is a significant source of stress for medical students and it is important we know how and where to direct them for support.

Medical students may lack motivation for a number of reasons. For example, some may simply not realise or want to participate in the amount of work involved, they may be over-confident in their abilities, or extra-curricular pursuits may prove more compelling than their coursework. Medical students worrying that they are studying the wrong course may e apprehensive about exploring this with their supervisors for fear of potential negative consequences.

How Do We Recognise When Students Are in Difficulty?

There is often a system in place within medical schools for alerting the block or placement lead for a student with ongoing difficulties so that extra support and/or monitoring may be put in place.

Unfortunately, the first sign that a student is in difficulty may be when they fail their end of year exam, a clinical placement, or some of their coursework. About 10% of students in each years' entrants to medical school will encounter academic failure at some stage in their programme (Holland, 2015), with a variety of factors contributing to this outcome.

Students in difficulty may present with apparent lapses in their professional behaviour or symptoms of illness, particularly mental illness. They may appear low, withdrawn, or anxious, or with any number of symptoms pertaining to ill health or excessive strain. Students may present in obvious distress or tell the supervisor of current or ongoing stressors. It is often an accumulation of low-level concerns, however, that signals that a student is in difficulty (General Medical Council, 2016b).

Aspects inherent to medical school curricula may lead to warning signs being missed – for example, changing placements every few weeks, lack of continuity of supervisors, and the numbers of students on placement. For this reason, it is important not to ignore or excuse a minor or one-off aberration without further exploration. Triangulation of student performance with other teachers on a clinical placement is advised. Medical schools are expected to have systems in place for collating and monitoring such concerns so that students with health or welfare issues can be identified and supported and so that unprofessional behaviour can be remediated early before it leads to more significant professionalism issues (General Medical Council, 2016b).

Box 7.1.1 What to Look Out For

- Persistent lateness
- Unprofessional appearance
- Appearing tired
- Smelling of alcohol or signs of intoxication
- Withdrawn
- Absence
- Coursework not submitted, late, or poorly completed
- Not able to answer questions
- Avoidant
- Rudeness
- Weepy
- Failure to respond to medical school communications

References

General Medical Council (2015). Supporting medical students with mental health conditions. https://medvle.buckingham.ac.uk/pluginfile.php/6630/mod_resource/content/1/Supporting_students_with_mental_health_conditions_0216.pdf_53047904.pdf (accessed 4 April 2022).

General Medical Council (2016a). Achieving good medical practice: guidance for medical students. www.gmc-uk.org/-/media/documents/achieving-good-medical-practice-20210722_pdf-66086678.pdf (accessed 4 April 2022).

General Medical Council (2016b). Professional behaviour and fitness to practise: guidance for medical schools and their students. www.gmc-uk.org/-/media/documents/professional-behaviour-and-fitness-to-practise-20210811_pdf-66085925.pdf (accessed 4 April 2022).

Holland, C. (2015). Critical review: Medical students' motivation after failure. *Advances in Health Sciences Education* **21**, 695–710.

O'Regan, A., Smithson, W. H., and Spain, E. (2018). Social media and professional identity: Pitfalls and potential. *Medical Teacher*, **40**, 112–16.

Ross, S., Cleland, J., and Macleod, M. J. (2006). Stress, debt and undergraduate medical student performance. *Medical Education* **40**, 584–9.

Schwenk, T. L., Davis, L., and Wimsatt, L. A. (2010). Depression, stigma, and suicidal ideation in medical students. *Journal of the American Medical Association*, **304** (11): 1181–90.

What Do I Do?

Dr Angela Cogan

Barriers to the Provision of Support

Unfortunately, students often present at crisis point, for example, having failed finals (Cleland et al., 2005), at a stage of having to take temporary withdrawal from the course, or with significant Fitness to Practise concerns. Late presentation of the student in difficulty is often due to a combination of student and teacher factors. By catching things early, student distress can be solved quickly, professionalism concerns can be remediated before it is too late, and students can learn to have confidence that 'it's okay not to be okay' so long as appropriate insight is demonstrated and help sought.

Teachers can be reluctant to raise concerns with their students. Issues that occur once or twice can be written off as transient. There can be over-empathising with the student experience and thus failure to discipline. Teachers can be fearful of reprisal from an angry student or they may worry about upsetting the student further (Brown et al., 2009). They may feel guilty if they have been unable to carry out a planned teaching session themselves notwithstanding a valid reason and thus excuse a student absence. Well-meaning but ultimately misguided teachers can over-support a struggling student, providing an abundance of assistance through academic hurdles rather than giving the student an objective appraisal of their current performance. It is essential, however, that doctors are honest and objective when assessing students for the benefit of the student and in the interest of patient safety (General Medical Council, 2014).

Medical students can be extremely reluctant to ask for help or support. They may think that they will be seen as weak or worry about breaches of confidentiality. They may have seen unhelpful behaviours role modelled and believe they should 'tough it out', or they may perceive that there will be negative consequences with respect to their future career. Sadly, there remains a huge amount of stigma regarding mental illness (Schwenk et al., 2010). Students may lack faith in the adequacy or availability of support services (Billingsley, 2015). Often a demanding schedule means students put off accessing support (Karp et al., 2018) and procrastinate until the situation becomes untenable.

How and When to Approach the Student in Difficulty

Owing to the variety of potential student issues, the multiple ways in which these present, and the relatively fleeting contact a teacher usually has with a medical student, it is worthwhile exploring any concerns regarding a student's academic or clinical performance, their affect, or their attitudes and behaviour. Problems identified early are often easier to solve and less severe, and it is important to consider if background factors are a main reason for the student's struggles.

Box 7.2.1 Raising Concerns in A Supportive Way

- Focus on the behaviour, not a trait
- As soon as possible after the occurrence
- At a suitable time, in a suitable place
- Supportive, non-judgemental
- Get the student's view
- Collaborative approach to problem solving

A framework for feedback is usually built into a clinical attachment and it is good to take advantage of this to provide a supportive environment for students. The initial meeting is useful for setting mutually agreed goals, but also for exploring with the students if they have any concerns. This gives the student the opportunity to share anything that may impact on their performance and provides an early opportunity to signpost the student to appropriate support or to make adjustments for support within the placement. Mid-point meetings are useful to discuss how things are going and to troubleshoot any issues while there is still time on the attachment. Students dislike hearing for the first time at the end-point assessment that there have been problems; however, if there are issues these must be raised, and it presents the chance to remediate and put supportive measures in place prior to future placements.

It is important to think about the time and place in which concerns are explored and the feedback given when approaching the student in difficulty. Concerns should be raised as soon as possible after an unhelpful behaviour or event has been observed, so that both supervisor and student can recall events accurately, and to allow the chance for remediation. Concerns should be discussed in a quiet and private place when interruption is unlikely, and the discussion should not feel rushed. Learners find it helpful if feedback focuses on strengths and weaknesses. Hewson and Little (1998) found that effective feedback is based on observations, given respectfully, clearly, and accurately, and with concern for the other's situation. Any feedback or discussion should be supportive and non-judgemental (Ende 1983); it is important to describe the behaviour rather than talk in terms of traits (Chowdhury et al., 2004): for example, 'I notice that you missed two ward rounds this week', rather than 'Your behaviour shows you are lazy and disinterested.' The process should be collaborative as far as possible to minimise the risk of defensiveness, humiliation or leaving the student feeling demoralised (Ende, 1983). The student should be given the chance to assess and give an explanation for the episode or situation and to suggest remedial measures, and it is important that the supervisor checks that both they and the student have the same understanding (Ramani et al., 2012) by, for example, asking the student to summarise the discussion.

How to Escalate Concerns in a Supportive Manner

Every medical school has support services for their students. Academics or clinicians involved in teaching students may not have direct knowledge or experience of these. It is important that all those involved in undergraduate medical education are aware of whom to contact to raise academic or pastoral concerns. Widespread measures include provision of personal tutors, pastoral support, and peer support. Those involved in providing pastoral care for students should not be involved in their assessment or progression to avoid conflict of interest. Students may confuse the role of their teacher, especially psychiatry supervisor, and expect treatment, rather than signposting. It is important for the teacher to avoid this, and to avoid over identification.

Students are often reluctant to attend support services due to concerns regarding confidentiality. Students will experience being privy to patient's medical information and will often need to be reassured that their own medical information will remain confidential unless a significant patient safety concern is raised.

Specific problems often require specialised services. Universities have learning development services to support students in developing their academic skills for the university environment – for example, in areas such as academic writing, critical thinking, study skills and time management. Often these services have individual and group sessions specifically aimed at the needs of medical students. Student financial services within universities provide financial support and advice and can help with access to hardship funds. Medical schools have access to their own bursaries and hardship funds, and student welfare services within each medical school can usually advise on these. Student Unions may provide access to financial, housing, and legal help or advocacy.

For students who are trying to cope with difficult personal and family circumstances, it sometimes helps for them to know that their supervisor, their pastoral care adviser, or someone else in the medical school is aware of this. They can help students by talking things over or signposting to outside help.

The majority of medical students will have sailed through their earlier educational experiences without too much effort. Medical students generally are not aware of and do not appreciate the hurdles, hardships, and failures their role models and teachers have endured (or are enduring) in their career journey. Failure is tough, as is tolerating the associated feelings of embarrassment or shame. Students can internalise a failure as a problem of a personal trait or ability rather than as a problem to be solved with attendant growth. This can be compounded in students with traits of perfectionism, anxiety, or low self-esteem. Medical schools often have well-being and resilience themes as a core part of their professionalism curriculum. Helping students cope with and learn from failure is a key role of any teacher, and referral to a medical school's internal pastoral support service can be helpful here.

Medical schools have a responsibility for student well-being and should create an environment in which mental health is openly discussed (General Medical Council, 2015). Students with mental health issues should be directed to their GP, who may refer them on to psychiatric services or to university counselling or psychological services. Students with any physical health issue should be directed to their GP. Students who are unwell may require time out for treatment and recovery from illness. Students with specific learning difficulties, ongoing mental or physical health issues, or other disabilities for which they require reasonable adjustment should register with university student disability services so that appropriate measures are put in place (General Medical Council, nd).

Insight about the nature and impact of illness is vital in relation to the student's fitness to practise. The GMC tells students that they must inform the medical school about any aspect of their health or personal circumstances that may affect their training or relationships with colleagues. Referral to the university's occupational health services for assessment is helpful if there is concern that a student's illness means they are not fit to practise. If a doctor who is involved in medical education has concerns about a student's fitness to practice it is essential that they inform the medical school. Medical schools have processes and structures to monitor and support students who have been identified as having specific problems. They also have procedures to investigate Fitness to Practise concerns and remediate if possible. Medical schools must provide students with pastoral support during this process.

Summary

Medical school can be an enjoyable and rewarding, but often stressful time for students. Adversity is a fact of life. Patient safety is of central concern. By supporting medical students through their ups and downs we can help them learn from their experiences and grow as professionals. It is essential that those teaching students are aware of why students might struggle, how this can present, and who to contact when extra support is required.

References

Billingsley, M. (2015). More than 80% of medical students with mental health issues feel under-supported. *BMJ*, **351**, h4521.

Brown, N. and Cooke, L. (2009). Giving effective feedback to psychiatric trainees. *Advances in Psychiatric Treatment*, **15**, 123–8.

Chowdhury, R. R. and Kalu, G. (2004). Learning to give feedback in medical education. *The Obstetrician & Gynaecologist*, **6**, 243–7.

Cleland, J., Arnold, R., and Chesser, A. (2005). Failing finals is often a surprise for the student but not the teacher: Identifying difficulties and supporting students with academic difficulties. *Medical Teacher*, **27**, 504–8.

Ende, J. (1983). Feedback in clinical medical education. *Journal of the American Medical Association*, **250**, 777–81.

General Medical Council (2014). Good Medical Practice. www.gmc-uk.org/ethical-guidance/ethical-guidance-for-doctors/good-medical-practice (accessed 4 April 2022).

General Medical Council (2015). Supporting medical students with mental health conditions. https://medvle.buckingham.ac.uk/pluginfile.php/6630/mod_resource/content/1/Supporting_students_with_mental_health_conditions_0216.pdf_53047904.pdf (accessed 4 April 2022).

General Medical Council (n.d.) Welcomed and valued: Supporting disabled learners in medical education and training. www.gmc-uk.org/education/standards-guidance-and-curricula/guidance/welcomed-and-valued/welcomed-and-valued-resources (accessed 4 April 2022).

Hewson, M. G. and Little, M. L. (1998). Giving feedback in medical education: verification of recommended techniques. *Journal of General Internal Medicine*, **13** (2): 111–16. https://doi.org/10.1046/j.1525-1497.1998.00027.x

Karp, J. and Levine, A. S. (2018). Mental health services for medical students – Time to act. *New England Journal of Medicine*, **379**, 13: 1196–8.

Ramani, S. and Krackov, S. K. (2012). Twelve tips for giving feedback effectively in the clinical environment. *Medical Teacher*, **34**, 787–791.

Schwenk, T. L., Davis, L., and Wimsatt, L. A. (2010). Depression, stigma, and suicidal ideation in medical students. *Journal of the American Medical Association*, **304**, (11): 1181–90.

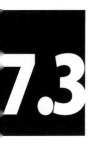

Raising Awareness and Promoting Well-Being

Dr Ahmed Hankir, Katharine Huggins, and Dr Rashid Zaman

Introduction

There is a growing body of evidence that suggests that mental health problems are over-represented in medical students. The prevalence of burnout, for example, in medical students is up to 71% greater than for the general population (Dyrbye et al., 2015; Tong, 2019). Moreover, a systematic review and meta-analysis on the mental health of medical students estimated that the prevalence of depression or depressive symptoms was 27.2% and suicidal ideation was 11.1% (Rotenstein et al., 2016). The duration and demands of the course, the intense and seemingly inflexible curriculum, regular assessments, and dysfunctional coping mechanisms (i.e. self-medication with alcohol and/or illicit substances) are some of the factors that might render medical students at increased risk of developing mental health problems (Erschens et al., 2018). Compounding the situation even further are the negative attitudes about mental health difficulties that are rampant in medical schools. Multiple studies have shown that stigma and 'a culture of shame' are formidable barriers to mental healthcare services; consequently, many medical students with mental health difficulties continue to suffer despite the availability of effective treatment (Grant, 2013; Dyrbye et al., 2015). In this book chapter we will explore these issues further and offer potential solutions.

Medical School Support Systems and Services

Historically, universities have recognised their responsibilities towards student well-being and endeavoured to provide support services (Givens and Tija, 2002; Hutchins 1964). Recognition of the importance of medical student well-being has led to the adoption and implementation of mental health policies such as investment in faculty training, promotion of independent pastoral services, and the devotion of time during student inductions to highlight support facilities (Grant, 2013).

The General Medical Council (GMC) found tutors teaching in small programmes took more informal and formal responsibility for providing pastoral student care (the nature of mental illness is such that it can deprive an individual of insight, and hence it may be that a tutor identifies a well-being concern before the student is self-aware). However, this individualised type of support is not available to every medical student, including already marginalised persons, such as those from Black, Asian, and Minority (BAME) backgrounds and those who identify with LGBTQ+ groups. Indeed, students have directly highlighted this as a cause for concern. For example, in March 2019 Goldsmiths University students occupied Deptford Town Hall in a protest requesting improved access to therapy for BAME students, and in October 2018 University College London students protested against the long waiting times for counselling (Shackle, 2019).

Although the impact of curricular differences, either systems-based or discipline-based on well-being remains unclear (Slavin, Schindler, and Chibnall, 2014), it is understood that progression through the medical course (Levine, Litwins, and Frye, 2006) and proximity of examinations negatively affects student's mental health (Radcliffe and Lester, 2003 Thiemann et al., 2020). Thus, a short-term benefit from, for example, an induction lecture on support services available may be rendered null when exam season arrives. It is therefore prudent, and often the case (Grant, 2013), for universities to reiterate well-being service closer to exams (e.g. provide 'booster sessions') and put in place targeted, proportionate and transparent support pathways for students.

No matter how accessible and extensive a support network is, however, it is rendered redundant if the medical school is unaware of student's problems. Weaknesses in the system, such as complex care processes for international students and students on clinical placements, may not be identified. Furthermore, as previously mentioned, ensuring consistency of support may vary dependant on the informal pastoral care students receive.

COVID-19 has presented further challenges in engendering student well-being Virtual classes allow education to continue relatively unhindered; however, in comparison to face-to-face classes, these are impersonal interactions. Students will have little opportunity to develop personal connections with their cohort and are therefore less likely to learn and be open about each other's stressors. Staff may also have greater difficulty in gauging warning signals. Student disengagement, non-attendance, and non cooperative behaviours are all warning signs of deterioration of a student's mental health Frustratingly, it is also these harbingers that may be stifled when student–staff interper sonal relationships are limited.

At present, universities acknowledge that mental health conditions are common and to be expected. However, students need reassurance that they can permit themselves to engage in the support pathways offered. Initiatives to further promote well-being must focus on prevention, access, quality, and positive experiences of care (Independent Mental Health Taskforce, 2016). For example, UCL monitors students' performance and uses the data as an early warning system and support cards that request the department to provide the student with reasonable adjustments. Here, the onus is taken off the student, and the process can alleviate some of the fear or embarrassment of repeatedly communicating about their concerns with tutors.

The promotion of mental health awareness is an important and effective primary health strategy. In order to fully support student well-being, universities need to adopt 'top-down and 'bottom-up' approaches that encourage bi-directional communication between student and faculty. Indeed, student mental health is a joint responsibility of both students and the medical school: students must take responsibility for looking after their health, and the university has an obligation to support them.

An example of a 'top-down approach' is equipping staff with the tools they need to identify early warning signs of psychological distress so that they can expeditiously mobilise a pathway for support between the student and pastoral services. It is imperative that this process is timely, transparent, and proportionate as early intervention is key for good outcomes (Givens and Tija, 2002). An example of a 'bottom-up' approach is communication from students to the university, which is more likely to occur at an earlier stage if there is an environment of trust, openness, and confidentiality regarding student self-referrals.

Mental Health-Related Stigma in Medical Schools

At present, stigma marginalises students, creates a major barrier to support, and is a corrosive force in the pursuit of good mental health. A 2010 study found that medical students engaged with self-stigmatisation by frequently agreeing that depressed students would be less respected and are less able to handle their responsibilities (Schwenk, Davis, and Wimsatt, 2010). Students who experience burnout are more likely to agree with stigma constructs such as personal weakness, public devaluation, and discrimination (Dyrbye et al., 2015).

The stigma of mental illness extends to a disparity in student empathy between pathologies. It is easy to develop empathy towards patients with a physical ailment such as breast cancer; however, a student may find it more difficult to do so for mental illness. Unconscious bias, micro-aggressions, and poor mental health literacy all contribute to the continuation of stigma and the negative caricatures they perpetuate. If difficulty in establishing empathy is a factor that preserves stigma in the medical profession, then the medical schools must create a representation of mental illness through which empathy can be developed. Representation could involve experiences with both patients and medical practitioners with a mental illness, creating an environment wherein mental health is spoken about freely and without fear of ramifications.

Experts by Personal and Professional Experience Anti-Stigma Programmes

The responsibility to enable students to build up trust in the support system lies with the university. Consistent with the prevailing stigma, medical practitioners rarely discuss their own experiences of coping with mental illness or their methods of promoting their mental well-being with the candour it demands. However, intergenerational transmission of stigma within medicine is not inevitable. Experts by Personal and Professional Experience (EPPE) and Medical School Psychiatry Societies ('Psych Socs') are resources that show promise in breaking the cycle of stigma (Pandian et al., 2020). As stated, developing empathy for a patient with a mental illness can be difficult for students with no experience of it; however, seeing senior physicians at the vanguard of the profession engaging with the topic pierces the bravado and shatters the illusion that doctors should be invincible (Harvey et al., 2009).

Case Study of an Expert by Personal and Professional Experience: 'The Wounded Healer'

In July 2006, when AH was a third-year medical student in Manchester, he woke up one morning to discover that his hometown in Lebanon had been bombed and that hundreds of people had been killed overnight. AH witnessed harrowing news reports containing images of dead bodies strewn on the streets of Lebanon and he was completely overwhelmed by the stress. AH subsequently developed a severe episode of psychological distress and was forced to interrupt his studies. However, debilitating though the symptoms of psychological distress were, the stigma was far worse. Instead of receiving care, empathy, and compassion, AH was ostracised, marginalised, and dehumanised by society, including by those who he thought were his closest companions. In his despair, AH developed suicidal ideation; however, he was able to resist the urge to act upon the impulses to end his own life since suicide is forbidden in Islam (Hankir et al., 2015). Fortunately (miraculously), AH eventu ally sought informal support from his Imam in his local mosque, who advised him to seek professional help from an NHS psychiatrist. AH received treatment, gradually recovered and resumed medical school with renewed resilience and determination. AH qualified from medical school in 2011 and he subsequently received the 2013 Royal College of Psychiatrists (RCPsych) Foundation Doctor of the Year and 2018 RCPsych Core Psychiatric Trainee of the Year Awards (the RCPsych awards mark the highest level of achievement in psychiatry in the United Kingdom).

AH noticed that when he was a medical student he didn't receive any teaching about the devastating effects of mental health-related stigma (this despite the fact that medical school has been described as a 'breeding ground' for mental health-related stigma; Thornicroft et al., 2007). AH thought this was a major problem since, as he knew only too well, stigma and 'a culture of shame' are formidable barriers to mental health services and consequently many medical students with mental health difficulties continue to suffer in silence despite the availability of effective treatment (Hankir et al., 2014).

AH urgently wanted to do something to reduce mental health stigma and discrimin ation. Any anti-stigma intervention must be evidence-based and data-driven. The Canadian Psychiatric Association reported that conventional education on mental illness alone does not reduce stigmatising attitudes and behaviours in medical students (Papish et al., 2013). Corrigan and colleagues conducted a systematic review and meta-analyses of outcome studies challenging the public stigma of mental illness and concluded that the most effective way of reducing mental health-related stigma in adults was through social contact with someone who has recovered from mental illness (Corrigan et al., 2012).

Equipped with this evidence, AH pioneered 'The Wounded Healer', an innovative anti stigma programme that blends the power of the performing arts and storytelling with psychiatry (Zaman et al., 2018). The Wounded Healer is a tripartite anti-stigma programme that incorporates elements of protest, education, and contact. The aims of the Wounded Healer are to engage, entertain, and educate to debunk the many myths about people with mental health difficulties, reduce mental health-related stigma, break down the barriers to mental health care, and encourage care-seeking (Zaman et al., 2018).

The Wounded Healer is a one-hour presentation that signposts AH's remarkable recovery from 'hopeless service user with mental illness' to RCPsych Award–winning doctor (Zaman et al., 2018). The Wounded Healer is delivered by an EPPE and therefore leverages the power of contact (Hankir et al., 2014). The Wounded Healer also contains all six key ingredients (one of which includes a personal testimony from a trained speaker who has lived experience of mental illness) identified by Stephanie Knaak and colleagues as necessary to reduce mental health-related stigma in healthcare providers (Knaak et al. 2014).

The Wounded Healer UK Lecture Circuit

A British study that recruited 302 students enrolled in medical schools throughout the United Kingdom revealed that 90% of respondents agreed or strongly agreed that a doctor with lived experience of a mental health condition should give a talk on medical student mental health (Hankir et al., 2014). AH has been fortunate to deliver The Wounded Healer to twenty-six out of the thirty-three medical school 'psych socs' (see Figure 7.3.1) through- out the United Kingdom (Zaman et al., 2018). The feedback that AH has received from

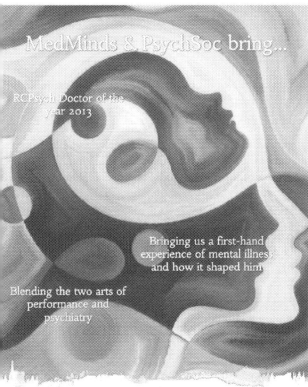

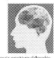

Figure 7.3.1 A flyer created by MedMinds and Birmingham Medical School Psychiatry Society to publicise The Wounded Healer event in Birmingham Medical Student. (Reproduced with permission from MedMinds and Birmingham Psych Soc.)

medical students about the Wounded Healer has been exceptionally positive. Below are some examples:

> Lectures like these should be given to all medical students to help reduce stigma and to encourage anyone struggling to get help. **Medical student, Sheffield**
>
> My friend tragically took his own life in January before your talk so I attended to seek answers that I came to realise that I'd never find, nonetheless I came out with something even better, peace of mind. I just wanted to let you know that what you do really does change peoples' lives. **Medical student, St George's University of London**

AH wished to scale up the number of people who could access The Wounded Healer. A multi-centre randomised controlled study revealed that film interventions have considerable and stable effects over time for stigma reduction and are highly scalable (Winkler et al., 2017).

AH collaborated with filmmakers from the London College of Communication and produced a film. *The Wounded Healer*, which has been digitised and screened at medical school. throughout the United Kingdom and beyond (Hankir et al., 2017).

Conclusion

Few medical students seek support for their well-being, and mental health-related stigma remains deeply entrenched in the medical culture. Medical schools must, therefore, pioneer innovative programmes that challenge mental health-related stigma and break down the barriers to mental healthcare services for students who urgently need them. Data derived from recent studies suggests that EPPEs can indeed reduce mental health-related stigma 91% of students who knew doctors obtained treatment for their mental health issues were more likely to access support themselves and 73% agreed that they would discuss concern. with doctors who had mental health problems and were open about their experience. (Martin et al., 2020). Although further research is imperative before scaling up anti stigma initiatives, medical schools now have a resource from which they can begin building programmes. Digitised film interventions would also be ideal to reduce mental health related stigma in medical schools since medical education is now largely being delivered online due to the COVID-19 pandemic.

References

Corrigan, P. W., Morris, S. B., Michaels, P. J., Rafacz, J. D., and Rüsch, N. (2012). Challenging the public stigma of mental illness: A meta-analysis of outcome studies. *Psychiatr Serv*, **63**, 963–73. Available at: https://pubmed .ncbi.nlm.nih.gov/23032675/ (accessed 10 Oct. 2020).

Dyrbye, L. and Shanafelt, T. (2015). A narrative review on burnout experienced by medical students and residents. *Medical Education*, **50** (1): 132–49. Available at: https://pubmed .ncbi.nlm.nih.gov/26695473/ (accessed 10 Oct. 2020).

Dyrbye, L. N., Eacker, A., Durning, S. J., et al. (2015). The impact of stigma and personal experiences on the help-seeking behaviors of medical students with burnout. *Academic Medicine*, **90** (7): 961–9. Available at: https:// pubmed.ncbi.nlm.nih.gov/25650824/ (accessed 10 Oct. 2020).

Erschens, R. S., Loda, T., Herrmann-Werner, A. et al. (2018). Behaviour-based functional and dysfunctional strategies of medical students to cope with burnout. ResearchGate, **23** (1): 1535738. Available at: www.researchgate .net/publication/328591259_Behaviour-based_functional_and_dysfunctional_

strategies_of_medical_students_to_cope_with_burnout (accessed 10 Oct. 2020).

Givens, J. L. and Tjia, J. (2002). Depressed medical students' use of mental health services. *Academic Medicine*, **77** (9): 918–21. Available at: https://journals.lww.com/academic medicine/Fulltext/2002/09000/Depressed_Medical_Students__Use_of_Mental_Health .24.aspx (accessed 10 Oct. 2020).

Grant, A., Rix, A., Mattick, K., Jones, D., and Winter, P. (2013). Identifying good practice among medical schools in the support of students with mental health concerns. Available at: www.gmc-uk.org/-/media/ documents/identifying-good-practice-among-medcal-schools-in-the-support-of-students-with-mental-healt-52884825.pdf (accessed 10 Oct. 2020).

Hankir, A., Carrick, F. R., Zaman, R. (2015). Islam, mental health and being a Muslim in the West. *Psychiatr Danub*. Sep; 27 Suppl 1, S53-9. Available at: https://pubmed .ncbi.nlm.nih.gov/26417737/ (accessed 10 Oct. 2020).

Hankir, A. K., Northall, A., Zaman, R. (2014). Stigma and mental health challenges in medical students. *BMJ Case Rep*. 2014 Sep 2 bcr2014205226. Available at: https://pubmed

.ncbi.nlm.nih.gov/25183806/ (accessed 10 Oct. 2020).

Iankir, A., Zaman, R., and Evans-Lacko, S. (2014). The Wounded Healer: An effective anti-stigma intervention targeted at the medical profession? *Psychiatr Danub.* Nov; 26 Suppl 1, 89–96. Available at: https://pubmed.ncbi.nlm.nih.gov/25413520/ (accessed 10 Oct. 2020).

Iankir, A., Zaman, R., Geers, B., et al. (2017). The Wounded Healer film: A London College of Communication event to challenge mental health stigma through the power of motion picture. *Psychiatr Danub.* Sep; 29 (Suppl 3): 307–312. Available at: https://pubmed.ncbi.nlm.nih.gov/28953783/ (accessed 10 Oct. 2020).

Iarvey, S. (2009). The Mental Health of Health Care Professionals. A review for the Department of Health Samuel B Harvey, Lecturer in Occupational Psychiatry Bee Laird, Postdoctoral Research Worker Max Henderson, Senior Lecturer in Occupational and Epidemiological Psychiatry. Available at: http://www.champspublichealth.com/writedir/8265The%20Mental%20Health%20of%20Health%20Care%20Professionals%20-%20A%20Review%20by%20the%20DH%20(June%202009).pdf (accessed 11 Oct. 2020).

Iutchins, E. (1964). The AAMC Longitudinal Study: Implications for medical education. *Academic Medicine*, 39 (3) 265–77. Available at: https://journals.lww.com/academicmedicine/Citation/1964/03000/The_AAMC_Longitudinal_Study__Implications_for.2.aspx (accessed 10 Oct. 2020).

Independent Mental Health Taskforce. (2016). Available at www.england.nhs.uk/mental-health/taskforce/ (accessed 4 April 2022).

Knaak, S. and Modgill, G. (2014). Patten SB: Key ingredients of antistigma programs for health care providers: A data synthesis of evaluative studies. *Can J Psychiatry*, 59 (10 Suppl 1), S19–26. Available at: https://pubmed.ncbi.nlm.nih.gov/25565698/ (accessed 10 Oct. 2020).

Levine, R. E., Litwins, S. D., and Frye, A. W. (2006). An evaluation of depressed mood in two classes of medical students. *Academic Psychiatry*, 30 (3): 235–7. Available at:

https://pubmed.ncbi.nlm.nih.gov/16728770/ (accessed 10 Oct. 2020).

Mahon, K. E., Henderson, M. K., and Kirch, D. G. Selecting tomorrow's physicians: The key to the future health care workforce. *Academic Medicine.* 2013; 88 (12): 1806–11. https://doi.org/10.097/ACM.0000000000000023. PMID: 2412862. Available at: https://pubmed.ncbi.nlm.nih.gov/24128626/ (accessed 10 Oct. 2020).

Martin, A., Chilton, J., Gothelf, D., and Amsalem, D. (2020). Physician self-disclosure of lived experience improves mental health attitudes among medical students: A randomized study. *Journal of Medical Education and Curricular Development*, 7. Available at: https://doi.org/10.1177/2382120519889352 (accessed 11 Oct. 2020).

Pandian, H., Mohamedali, Z., Chapman, G. E., et al. (2020). Psych Socs: Student-led psychiatry societies, an untapped resource for recruitment and reducing stigma. *BJPsych Bulletin*, 44 (3): 91–5. Available at: https://doi.org/10.1192/bjb.2019.88 (accessed 11 Oct. 2020).

Papish, A., Kassam, A., Modgill, G., Vaz, G., Zanussi, L., and Patten, S. (2013). Reducing the stigma of mental illness in undergraduate medical education: A randomized controlled trial. *BMC Med Educ*, 13 (141). Available at: https://pubmed.ncbi.nlm.nih.gov/24156397/ (accessed 10 Oct. 2020).

Radcliffe, C. and Lester, H. (2003). Perceived stress during undergraduate medical training: A qualitative study. *Medical Education*, 37 (1): 32–8. Available at: https://pubmed.ncbi.nlm.nih.gov/12535113/ (accessed 10 Oct. 2020).

Rotenstein, L. S., Ramos, M. A., Torre, M., et al. (2016). Prevalence of depression, depressive symptoms, and suicidal ideation among medical students. *JAMA*, 316 (21): 2214. Available at: https://pubmed.ncbi.nlm.nih.gov/27923088/ (accessed 10 Oct. 2020).

Schwenk, T. L., Davis, L., and Wimsatt, L. A. (2010). Depression, stigma, and suicidal ideation in medical students. *JAMA*, 304 (11): 1181. Available at: https://jamanetwork.com/

journals/jama/fullarticle/186586 (accessed 11 Oct. 2020).

Shackle, S. (2019). 'The way universities are run is making us ill': Inside the student mental health crisis. *The Guardian*. Available at: www.theguardian.com/society/2019/sep/27/anxiety-mental-breakdowns-depression-uk-students (accessed 11 Oct. 2020).

Slavin, S. J., Schindler, D. L., and Chibnall, J. T. (2014). Medical student mental health 3.0. *Academic Medicine*, **89** (4): 573–7. Available at: www.ncbi.nlm.nih.gov/pmc/articles/PMC4885556/ (accessed 11 Oct. 2020).

Thiemann, P., Brimicombe, J., Benson, J., and Quince, T. (2020). When investigating depression and anxiety in undergraduate medical students timing of assessment is an important factor: A multicentre cross-sectional study. *BMC Medical Education*, **20** (1). Available at: www.ncbi.nlm.nih.gov/pmc/articles/PMC7181528/ (accessed 10 Oct. 2020).

Thornicroft, G., Rose, D., Kassam, A., and Sartorius, N. (2007). Stigma: Ignorance, prejudice or discrimination? *Br J Psychiatry*.

Mar; **190**, 192–3. Available at: https://pubmed.ncbi.nlm.nih.gov/17329736/ (accessed 10 Oct. 2020).

Tong, G. (2019). World Mental Health Day 2018, but how aware are medical students?. *Advances in Medical Education and Practice* Volume **10**, 217–19. Available at: www.ncbi.nlm.nih.gov/pmc/articles/PMC6524131/ (accessed 10 Oct. 2020).

Winkler, P., Janoušková, M., Kožený, J., et al. (2017). Short video interventions to reduce mental health stigma: a multi-centre randomised controlled trial in nursing high schools. *Soc Psychiatry Psychiatr Epidemiol*. Dec; **52** (12): 1549–57. Available at: https://pubmed.ncbi.nlm.nih.gov/29101447/ (accessed 10 Oct. 2020).

Zaman, R., Carrick, F. R., and Hankir, A. (2018). Innovative approaches to improving the image of psychiatrists and psychiatry amongst medical students and doctors in the UK. *Psychiatr Danub*. Nov; **30** (Suppl 7) 616–19. Available at: https://pubmed.ncbi.nlm.nih.gov/30439859/ (accessed 10 Oct. 2020).

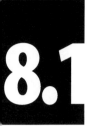

Getting Involved

Dr Neera Gajree

Introduction

Mental illness is common and therefore all doctors will regularly encounter patients suffering from mental health problems (Dale, Bhavsar, and Bhugra, 2007). Consequently, delivering high-quality undergraduate psychiatry teaching is essential to the future provision of holistic patient care (Royal College of Psychiatrists, n.d.).

The General Medical Council (2013) states that the teaching and training of doctors and students is a core requirement of all medical staff. The curricula created by the Royal College of Psychiatrists (2020, 2022) for both core and higher specialist training highlight the need for all trainee psychiatrists to deliver education. As such, trainees must be able to evidence involvement in teaching at their Annual Review of Competence Progression (ARCP).

Psychiatry trainees play a crucial role in undergraduate teaching. Although consultant psychiatrists usually take responsibility for providing educational supervision to medical students, the day-to-day job of teaching medical students is often delegated to trainees (Vassilas et al., 2003). In fact, a number of studies suggest that psychiatry trainees are the primary educator of students (Hickie, Nash, and Kelly, 2013; Bing-You and Sproul, 1992). Students often prefer trainee-led teaching to that delivered by senior clinicians (Thampy et al., 2019), and the teaching delivered by trainees to students can be considered as 'near peer'. 'Near peer' teaching occurs when teachers are at least one year senior to their learners (de Menzes and Premnath, 2016). Given their closeness in stage, trainee psychiatrists may be more familiar with the training requirements of students, the nature of university examinations, and what concerns or worries students might have about psychiatry.

Why Should I Get Involved in Teaching?

Teaching medical students can have a number of benefits for psychiatry trainees. As trainees have less knowledge than consultants, teaching can be a powerful motivator for self-directed learning and can lead to improved knowledge acquisition (Weiss and Needlman, 1998). The requirement to teach students can highlight gaps in trainees' knowledge, which can stimulate learning (Painter, Rodenhauser, and Rudisill, 1987). In a survey by Korszun and colleagues (2011) 99% of psychiatry trainees agreed that they were interested in teaching medical students. If it is an activity they find enjoyable, teaching can also contribute to trainees' job satisfaction (Apter, Metzger, and Glassroth, 1988). Undergraduate teaching requires a number of skills, including patience, adaptability, communication skills, appraisal skills, examination skills, and motivation for learning. Many of these skills are transferable to clinical practice and are necessary for maintaining lifelong professional development.

However, teaching can cause anxiety in trainees who don't feel skilled in this area. Although teaching is a responsibility usually given to trainees, they may lack formal training in how to teach (Hickie, Nash, and Kelly, 2013; Bramble, 1991). Most psychiatry trainees believe that all doctors involved in undergraduate teaching should receive training in educational methods (Korszun et al., 2011). As such, there are a number of options available to trainees who wish to develop their teaching skills, including 'Teach the Teacher' courses run by various institutions and online CPD modules (including one provided by the Royal College of Psychiatrists). At present, there is no requirement for psychiatry trainees in the United Kingdom to undertake training in medical education and doing so requires motivation, time, and often funding. It is therefore important for trainees to discuss their teaching commitments with their consultants in order to receive adequate support.

Psychiatry trainees have identified a lack of knowledge about what topics to teach and insufficient knowledge of students' learning objectives as further difficulties associated with undergraduate teaching (Swainson, Marsh, and Tibbo, 2010; Kates and Lesser, 1985). It would be beneficial for university learning objectives for psychiatry to be disseminated to all medical staff involved in educating students so that they are better guided on what to teach.

How to Get Involved

There are a number of ways for psychiatry trainees to get involved in teaching. Trainees may wish to start contributing to ad hoc, informal teaching at a local level, and work up to giving lectures as they gain confidence and experience.

Medical student inductions are a good place to start. These are often organised by NHS boards or trusts but trainees can also play an integral role in inducting students to their placements. The General Medical Council (2011) states that undergraduate clinical placement inductions should include familiarisation with placement settings, briefing students on the rules and procedures of placements and introducing students to relevant staff members. Trainees can help orient students by assisting with these tasks. Trainees can also assist students in developing learning objectives for their time in psychiatry and help plan available learning opportunities to help meet these objectives. By identifying areas of psychiatry that students are interested in and facilitating experiences in these areas, trainees can help to enhance the value and enjoyability of placements for students.

Once students are up and running in their psychiatry placement, there will be plenty of opportunities for informal teaching as they shadow trainees and their team. Trainees have a range of clinical commitments which can provide valuable teaching opportunities. By demonstrating how to assess and manage patients, trainees can teach students through modelling, which Stalmeijer and colleagues (2008) noted can enhance learning in clinical practice. It is important that patient consent is always sought if students are present.

Multidisciplinary ward rounds can be very educational for students. El-Sayeh and colleagues (2006) highlighted the importance of allowing specific time in ward rounds to discuss and explain management issues. Trainees can play a role in ensuring that students are actively included in discussions, and in explaining unfamiliar terms or concepts.

Students should gain experience of assessing inpatients more independently in psychiatry wards. Trainees are often best placed to teach important 'on the ground' issues required for this, such as interview safety and how to interact with and talk to patients. Students should be encouraged to assess the mental health of patients and present their findings. Trainees can give feedback to students on their skills in history-taking and mental state examination, provide focussed teaching, and complete assessments.

Students may also attend clinics and even shadow trainees during on-call shifts if they re very keen. Earlier chapters in this book explore how you might make the most of eaching in these clinical settings (see Chapter 3.2).

ormal Teaching

n many areas, formal teaching for students is provided by Higher Trainees, who have obtained their MRCPsych qualification and thus have a broad psychiatry knowledge base. Teaching may be organised both within psychiatry placements and at universities.

Teaching students on psychiatry placements usually involves teaching small groups as psychiatric hospitals are limited by the number of students that they can accommodate at one time. Teaching at universities often involves teaching larger numbers of students ogether. Formal teaching can occur in a number of ways including the following, and hese are explored separately in Chapters 4.1, 4.2, and 4.4 of this book.

Bedside Teaching

Trainees may wish to undertake bedside teaching, whereby they teach students in the presence of patients. Students mostly perceive bedside teaching in psychiatry to be useful, out to a lesser extent than in other more practical specialities (Indraratna et al., 2013). Although bedside teaching confers advantages to students such as facilitating the development of clinical reasoning skills and bedside manner, it has declined in popularity over ecent years for a number of reasons, including its time-consuming nature and the willingness of patients to participate (Qureshi and Maxwell, 2012; Indraratna, Greenup, and Yang, 2013). Trainees will need to consider these factors if teaching in this way.

Tutorials

Trainees can facilitate the discussion of topics related to mental health during small group tutorials. As students may be less intimidated by trainees, they may be more likely to express worries or ask questions during small-group teaching (Stewart and Feltovich, 1988). Some topics end themselves better to teaching through tutorials than other means, such as stigma in mental health.

Simulation

Simulation, which can be defined as educational activities that replicate clinical scenarios, is increasingly used as a means of teaching students (Al-Elq, 2010). Trainees can simulate patients presenting with various mental health disorders and ask students to assess them. Due to their breadth of experience and knowledge, it is likely that many Higher Trainees will be able to portray patients with mental illness in a more sensitive and realistic manner. Mavis and colleagues (2006) noted that students found feedback from staff who simulated patients useful in improving their skills.

Lectures

Lectures are commonly used to teach larger groups of undergraduate students in psychiatry. Universities can at times struggle to get busy NHS consultants to deliver lectures, and Higher Trainees may wish to contact their local university's psychiatry subdean to enquire about available teaching opportunities. In order to enhance the learning of students, it i important for lecturers to identify the key messages that they wish to convey, ensure that th material is covered in a logical structure, and enrich it with information that cannot b obtained from textbooks, such as personal experience (Long and Lock, 2014). The lectur should conclude with a summary of the main points, further sources of information, an enough time for questions.

Beyond Undergraduate Teaching

Although this book is focussed on undergraduate psychiatry teaching, it is worth noting th opportunities available for Higher Trainees to teach a wider range of medical colleagues.

Higher Trainees can provide near-peer teaching to other postgraduate doctors i training. Given that most Higher Trainees have recently been Core Trainees, the experienc and knowledge they can share with colleagues can be valuable. Teaching opportunitie include providing part of the junior doctor induction, delivering lectures to junior doctor at regional teaching programmes, and teaching examination skills to Core Trainees prepar ing for MRCPsych examinations.

Higher Trainees can also get involved in providing mental health-related teaching t doctors working in other specialities (e.g. Accident and Emergency, Obstetrics an Gynaecology, etc.). The UK Foundation Programme Curriculum (2016) includes compe tencies related to mental health. Thus, there may be opportunities to teach groups o Foundation Year doctors, and Higher Trainees may wish to contact the local Foundatio Programme Director to discuss this. Many general hospitals run weekly 'Grand Round educational programmes for all physicians that are often hosted by different specialties o a rotating basis. Higher Trainees may consider contacting whoever organises this pro gramme to enquire about providing psychiatry related teaching there.

Conclusion

Psychiatry Trainees play an important part in undergraduate teaching. Teaching is largel viewed as an enjoyable component of a psychiatry trainee's job and can be very valuable t students. However, it is also important that trainees receive appropriate training an supervision for this important role. There are numerous opportunities for trainees to ge involved in educating students – for example at induction, during clinical work, an through providing formal teaching. Higher Trainees in psychiatry may also expand thei teaching to the education of other doctors.

References

Al-Elq, H. A. (2010). Simulation-based medical teaching and learning. *Journal of Family and Community Medicine*, **17**, 35–40.

Apter, A., Metzger, R., and Glassroth, J. (1988). Residents' perceptions of their role as teachers. *Journal of Medical Education*, **63**, 900–5.

Bing-You, R. G. and Sproul, M. S. (1992). Medical students' perceptions of themselves and residents as teachers. *Medical Teacher*, **14**, 133–8.

Bramble, D. J. (1991). 'Teaching the teachers' – a survey of trainees' teaching experience. *Psychiatric Bulletin*, **15**, 751–2.

Dale, J. T., Bhavsar, V., and Bhugra, D. (2007). Undergraduate medical education of Psychiatry in the West. *Indian Journal of Psychiatry*, **49**, 166–98.

Menezes, S. and Premnath, D. (2016). Near-peer education: a novel teaching program. *International Journal of Medical Education*, **30**, 160–7.

-Sayeh, H., Budd, S., Waller, R., et al. (2006). How to win the hearts and minds of students in psychiatry. *Advances in Psychiatric Treatment*, **12**, 182–92.

eneral Medical Council. (2011). Clinical placements for medical students. Available at: www.gmc-uk.org/-/media/documents/Clinical_placements_for_medical_students__guidance_0815.pdf_56437824.pdf (accessed 10 September 2020).

eneral Medical Council. (2013). Good medical practice. Available at: www.gmc-uk.org/ethical-guidance/ethical-guidance-for-doctors/good-medical-practice (accessed 4 April 2022).

ickie, C., Nash, L., and Kelly, B. (2013). The role of trainees as clinical teachers of medical students in psychiatry. *Australasian Psychiatry*, **21**, 583–6.

draratna, P. L., Greenup, L. C., and Yang, T. X. (2013). Bedside teaching in Australian clinical schools: A national study. *Journal of Biomedical Education*, 948651. Available from: https://doi.org/10.1155/2013/948651 (accessed 10 September 2020).

ates, N. S. and Lesser, A. L (1985). The resident as a teacher: A neglected role. *Canadian Journal of Psychiatry*, **30**, 418–21.

orszun, A., Dharmaindra, N., Koravangattu, V., et al. (2011). Teaching medical students and recruitment to psychiatry: Attitudes of psychiatric clinicians, academics and trainees. *The Psychiatrist*, **35**, 350–3.

ong, A. and Lock, B. (2014). Lectures and large groups. In Swanwick, T. (ed.) *Understanding Medical Education: Evidence, Theory and Practice*. 2nd ed. Chichester: John Wiley & Sons, 137–48.

avis, B., Turner, J., Lovell, K., et al. (2006). Faculty, students, and actors as standardized patients: Expanding opportunities for performance assessment. *Teaching and Learning in Medicine*, **18**, 130–6.

Painter, A. F., Rodenhauser, P. R., and Rudisill, J. R. (1987). Psychiatric residents as teachers: A national survey. *Journal of Psychiatric Education*, **11**, 21–6.

Qureshi, Z. and Maxwell, S. (2012). Has bedside teaching had its day? *Advances in Health Sciences Education*, **17**, 301–4.

Royal College of Psychiatrists. (2010). A Competency Based Curriculum for Specialist Training in Psychiatry. Available at: www.rcpsych.ac.uk/docs/default-source/training/curricula-and-guidance/general_psychiatry_curriculum_march_2019.pdf?sfvrsn=9e53c99a_6 (accessed 10 September 2020).

Royal College of Psychiatrists. (2013). A Competency Based Curriculum for Specialist Core Training in Psychiatry. Available at: www.rcpsych.ac.uk/docs/default-source/training/curricula-and-guidance/core_psychiatry_curriculum_may_2019.pdf?sfvrsn=f8594b3e_6 (accessed 10 September 2020).

Royal College of Psychiatrists. (n.d.). Supporting medical students. Available at: www.rcpsych.ac.uk/become-a-psychiatrist/supporting-medical-students (accessed 4 April 2022).

Royal College of Psychiatrists. (2020). A Competency Based Curriculum for Specialist Core Training in Psychiatry. Available at: www.rcpsych.ac.uk/training/curricula-and-guidance/curricula-implementation/draft-core-psychiatry-curriculum (accessed 4 April 2022).

Royal College of Psychiatrists. (2022). Higher Speciality Curricula 2022. Available at:www.rcpsych.ac.uk/training/curricula-and-guidance/curricula-implementation/draft-higher-specialty-curricula-2022 (accessed 4 April 2022).

Stalmeijer, R. E., Dolmans, D., Wolfhagen, I., et al. (2008). Cognitive apprenticeship in clinical practice: Can it stimulate learning in the opinion of students? *Advances in Health Sciences Education*, **14**, 535–46.

Stewart, D. E. and Feltovich, P. J. (1988). Why residents should teach: The parallel process of teaching and learning. In Edwards, J. C.

and Marrier R. L. (eds.) *Clinical Teaching for Medical Residents: Roles, Techniques and Programs*. New York: Springer, pp. 3–14.

Swainson, J., Marsh., M., and Tibbo, P. G. (2010). Psychiatric residents as teachers: development and evaluation of a teaching manual. *Academic Psychiatry*, **34**, 305–9.

Thampy, H., Alberti, H., Kirkchuk, L., et al. (2019). Near peer teaching in general practice. *British Journal of General Practice*, **69**, 12–13.

The UK Foundation Programme Curriculum (2016). The Foundation Programme Curriculum 2016. Available at: https://foundationprogramme.nhs.uk/curriculum/ (accessed 4 April 2022).

Vassilas, C. A., Brown, N., Wall, D., et al. (2003). 'Teaching the teachers' in psychiatry. *Advances in Psychiatric Treatment*, **9**, 308–1.

Weiss, V. and Needlman, R. (1998). To teach i to learn twice: Resident teachers learn more *Archives of Pediatrics and Adolescent Medicine*, **152**, 190–2.

8.2

Formal Roles in Medical Education

Dr Wai Lan Imrie

Teaching is an integral part of being a good doctor (GMC, 2013: domain 3). The Royal College of Psychiatrists has included teaching as a requirement and intended learning outcome (ILO) for core training and subspecialties (e.g. Core curriculum; RCP, 2020, p. 59). Therefore, there is an expectation that every doctor should be required to educate not just future doctors, but also other health professionals, and not least the patients with whom we come into contact.

However, throughout the course of your medical training there are some key people who are responsible for organising, delivering, and ensuring the quality of your training programmes. The aim of this chapter is to make you more aware of these roles, and the possible future career opportunities for those of you who have an interest in medical education and how this can be developed.

Trainees are often surprised to learn that many formal medical education roles do not require additional formal teaching qualifications and are not essential for career progression. However, postgraduate medical education qualifications are undoubtedly helpful for personal development and for gaining an understanding of different teaching and learning theories and techniques. This may be useful in developing a new programme or improving struggling programmes. In common with most aspects of medicine, experiential learning is crucial for these roles. Genuine enthusiasm, an interest in medical education, and having good organisational skills are essential qualities. The skills required to be a good doctor are also pertinent to being a good educator: for example, good communication skills and team working. Often these roles are filled by consultants who, as trainees, have shown a keen interest in medical education, have sought opportunities to get involved in teaching, and go on to further develop these interests in their consultant careers.

Knowing the right people in your university and training programme is key to getting the right experience and developing a network. As with most career progression, being in the right place at the right time and having the relevant skills when an opportunity presents itself is vital. You will find that a training programme with a reputation for being well organised and with good systems in place is likely to attract more applicants and thus there will be more competition for vacant posts. The posts are advertised within the university, deanery and local education providers (LEPs) in open competition. Some roles are time-limited and post holders may have to reapply for the post when their original period of appointment expires. For the purposes of this chapter, GMC terms will be used where possible. Some roles will require candidates to be recognised as trainers by the GMC (GMC, 2012, p. 15). Only roles where no additional postgraduate medical qualifications are necessary and to which any jobbing psychiatrist can aspire will be discussed.

University and Undergraduate Roles

Each medical school will have slightly different systems and structures, but, broadl speaking, the equivalent roles listed here will be found in each school. The teaching o undergraduates in preclinical years is usually conducted by non-clinical staff in the medical faculty from human science backgrounds: for example, lecturers and professor in physiology, anatomy, biochemistry, etc. As would be expected, clinicians are respon sible for teaching in the clinical years and heads of year can be from any medica specialty. Ultimately, the GMC has oversight of the educational governance of ever medical school. There are several roles that require the post holder to be recognised a a trainer; these are identified under each role as described herein (GMC, 2012, p. 15)

Clinical Lecturer

As a trainee this may be the first opportunity to become involved in teaching in a mor formal way. Trainees who have a talent for and an interest in research could conside such posts. Clinical lecturer posts allow trainees to have protected time for researc whilst at the same time completing training in their specialty. Most specialist pro grammes will require that you hold a national training number before being eligible t apply. The proportion of clinical and research sessions within the working week will var from programme to programme and may require an extension of your certificate o completion of training (CCT). Within these posts there is opportunity to teach under graduates and other allied health professionals through the university. Some clinica lecturers will take time out of the programme to concentrate on research and obtainin additional postgraduate qualifications (such as a PhD) before returning to and complet ing their training and obtaining their CCT. Post-CCT clinical lecturers can develop i two main directions. They may continue with research and continue as clinical lecturer with honorary consultant psychiatry status within the NHS. This requires that there i a substantive clinical lecturer post at the university. Most trainees who have been clinica lecturers apply for consultant psychiatrists' posts and continue their research within thei clinical role.

Honorary Clinical Lecturer

Any trainee in higher specialty training, specialty grade posts, or a consultant role is eligibl to apply for honorary lecturer status as long as they can provide evidence of involvement i teaching or research. This application has to be supported by the appropriate subdean o senior lecturer for psychiatry at the medical school and will require approval by the senio training committee within the university medical faculty. Most clinical lectures for th undergraduate course are delivered by honorary clinical lecturers. There is no direc remuneration attached to roles, but this status carries some perks, for example the use o university facilities such as libraries and gyms.

Educational Supervisors for Undergraduates

These are jobbing psychiatrists – consultants and specialty grade doctors who undertak the day-to-day supervision of medical students on their clinical placements. They shoul have time assigned in their job plans to allow for this and need to be recognised a trainers.

Postgraduate Tutors

This is usually an educational supervisor who has been appointed by the LEP to coordinate undergraduate clinical placements and local teaching. These posts are often a stepping-stone to other medical educator roles. The postgraduate tutors liaise closely with the hospital subdean.

Hospital Subdean for Psychiatry

Each medical school will have a hospital subdean (or equivalent) who is responsible for the organisation of psychiatric hospital medical student placements and delivering teaching programmes to fulfil curriculum requirements. The psychiatry subdean (depending on the university) has responsibility for organisation of centralised teaching of undergraduates. In larger programmes, individual placements within psychiatric hospitals may be delegated to postgraduate tutors. Hospital subdeans will have time negotiated in their job plans or additional sessions agreed.

Heads of Year at Medical School

There is a head of year for each medical school year. The preclinical heads are usually appointed from the university medical science lecturers and professors and are not usually involved in clinical work. The heads of year for clinical years are usually clinicians who have been involved in research, lecturing, and teaching in the undergraduate course. They will have sessional time within their job plans negotiated for this. They are responsible for overseeing the progress of students in their year and work closely with hospital subdeans in each specialty.

Deanery and Postgraduate Roles

The educational governance of core and specialist psychiatric training programmes is the purview of the Royal College, GMC, local deaneries, and Director of Medical Education (DME)s. The curriculum for each programme is set by the college, and is ultimately approved by the GMC and delivered to high standards by the local deaneries. In addition, LEPs will employ a director of medical education who will be responsible for the recognition of trainers, and who will also ensure that the service is able to deliver the training to a high and consistent quality. This requires sophisticated and necessary interaction between these organisations to ensure that training programmes attain and retain their quality and standards of education. The infrastructure within each deanery will be similar and there are many key positions to which a budding educationalist can aspire. For the purposes of this chapter, the possibilities that lie within your local LEP will be outlined. These roles also can lead to further opportunities within the Royal College.

Named Clinical Supervisors

As defined by the GMC, a clinical supervisor 'is a trainer who is responsible for overseeing a specified trainee's clinical work throughout a placement' (GMC, 2012, p. 18). Within psychiatry, broadly speaking, an apprenticeship teaching and learning model has been retained. As such, the named clinical supervisor will usually be the consultant with whom the trainee has been placed. In some services the post may be split, in which case one of the consultants will be a named supervisor; this person will be responsible for delivering the one-hour educational supervision to the trainee and will have time in their job plan specifically for this. Most consultants will need to be recognised as a named clinical supervisor if they are allocated trainees on a regular basis.

Named Educational Supervisors

A named educational supervisor 'is a trainer who is selected and appropriately trained to be responsible for the overall supervision and management of a trainee's trajectory of learning and educational progress during a placement or series of placements' (GMC, 2012, p. 18)

In core training there may be several educational supervisors in the programme – this largely depends on the size and number of LEPs in the programme. These roles are usually appointed by the LEP through competitive interview if there is more than one candidate. Core educational supervisors are usually responsible for the organisation of internal teaching and ensuring Core Trainees are prepared for their Annual Review of Competency to Progress (ARCP). There may be additional sessional payment or time in their job plan to allow for the additional work this requires. Similar structures exist in higher training depending on the size and geographical spread of LEPS within each programme. Most named educational supervisors will also be named clinical supervisors.

Training Programme Directors

Training programme directors (TPDs) are appointed by the deanery to manage and oversee the training programme. They are appointed through open competition via the LEPs. They have responsibility for the placement of the trainees in the programme and will liaise with educational supervisors in the larger programme to coordinate trainee placements. They are instrumental in organising and delivering the ARCP for every trainee in their programme and will have additional sessions in their job plan for this role.

Associate Postgraduate Dean for Psychiatry

The associate postgraduate dean for psychiatry (APGD) will oversee all the psychiatric specialties and have management responsibilities for their TPDs in their region/deanery. They liaise closely with the Royal College, GMC, and DMEs, reporting back to the dean. Sessional time is allocated.

Dean of Psychiatry

Within each deanery there will be a dean of psychiatry overseeing the whole programme. They will not necessarily be a psychiatrist – this is dependent on the deanery management structures. Currently, in the Scotland deanery, the dean of psychiatry has a background in Obstetrics and Gynaecology.

Director of Medical Education and Deputies

The director of medical education (DME) is employed by the LEP to ensure that the quality of training for undergraduates and postgraduates meets GMC standards. They are responsible for ensuring that there is a process for recognising trainers in each LEP. They provide an additional layer of scrutiny and educational governance for trainees. DMEs and deputies usually have a background in medical education, as knowledge of training structures is helpful in this role. They liaise closely with the service managers as well as the medical educators to ensure that the balance between service provision and training is achieved for trainees.

Conclusion

There is a raft of opportunities for any clinician who is interested in medical education, none of which require any formal postgraduate qualification, though some will require you to be a recognised trainer. These roles are often rewarding and there is satisfaction in knowing that you have contributed to the education and development of future generations of psychiatrists.

Anyone who is interested in these roles is advised to show willingness at the earliest opportunity, for example during higher specialist training. Seeking out the relevant people in your LEP or university and getting involved is a helpful first step. Existing educators are likely to be receptive to offers of help. When you take up your substantive post, further opportunities are likely to arise over time. Clear expressions of interest and evidence of related expertise and experience, along with enthusiasm, will be helpful in securing these additional opportunities.

References

General Medical Council (2012). Recognising and Approving Trainers: The implementation plan. Available at: www.gmc-uk.org/-/media/documents/approving-trainers-implementation-plan-aug-12-v2_pdf-661442 33 (accessed 16 October 2020).

General Medical Council (2013). Good Medical Practice Domain 3: Communication partnership and teamwork. Available at: www.gmc-uk.org/ethical-guidance/ethical-guidance-for-doctors/good-medical-practice/domain-3---communication-partnership-and-teamwork (accessed 4 April 2022).

Royal College of Psychiatrists (2020). A Competency Based Curriculum for Specialist Core Training in Psychiatry. Available at: www.rcpsych.ac.uk/training/curricula-and-guidance/curricula-implementation/draft-core-psychiatry-curriculum (accessed 4 April 2022).

Training in Medical Education

8.3

Dr Amy Manley

Why Train in Medical Education?

For centuries, teaching has been part of the role of the doctor. With little formal educational training, doctors learnt how to teach on-the-job. Educational theory and research were used infrequently, with doctors basing their teaching style on that which they experienced and learning from how students responded. In recent decades, formal training and qualification in medical education has become increasingly available and popular. Certificates in medical education are frequently cited in the desirable criteria of educational roles.

What Training is Available?

Training in how to teach is available for doctors across the United Kingdom and further afield. Courses vary from region to region and are targeted at different levels of training. Courses can be broadly divided into accredited courses, which lead to a degree (or credit towards a degree) and those which don't. Most people start with the latter; these offer the opportunity to develop specific educational skills without the financial commitment or assessment requirements expected at degree level. If you are looking for some key ways to improve your teaching or assessment of students, it would be well worth investigating such courses. Degree-level courses allow you to look deeper into the theoretical underpinnings of medical education, and help you reflect on your practice and critically appraise the evidence base. You can apply both your theoretical and practical degree learning to your practice whether you want to develop assessments, creative ways of teaching, or a curriculum. Having a degree in medical education may also be a requirement for some jobs.

Non-Degree Teaching Courses: 'Train the Trainer' Courses

Teaching is a necessary competency to complete core and higher psychiatry training, and many psychiatrists choose to complete courses in teaching in order to develop workplace and formal teaching skills. Such courses are often very practical, focussing on ways to improve teaching or develop new teaching methods, for example group facilitation or Objected Structured Clinical Examination (OSCE). Face-to-face courses often involve practical experiences such as the opportunity to examine a mock OSCE or get feedback on a micro-teaching session. This can be invaluable when looking to develop a specific applied skill. Other teaching sessions focussing on the underpinning knowledge of medical education can also be valuable to inform broader education practice. A huge part of developing skills in medical education comes from observing, learning from others, and discussing your own experiences, therefore group discussion with like-minded participants can allow you to develop novel solutions to challenges you may face. Some courses are elivered online and try to emulate a face-to-face setting, with opportunities for small group earning facilitated remotely.

University medical schools, Health Education England (HEE) Local Education and Training Boards and NHS Trust medical education departments offer training for clinicians involved in teaching their students or interested in taking on teaching roles e.g. OSCE examiner). Many of these are free and lead to additional local teaching opportunities, such as becoming a Problem Based Learning (PBL) facilitator. Some can even contribute to degree credit, should you wish to take them further. You will also meet like-minded colleagues (often with multidisciplinary backgrounds) and tutors, who can be a great source of further information about medical education opportunities and courses.

For more information about local training and roles in medical education, speak to the following people or check out their websites:

- Your HEE Local Education Training Board (LETB) or School of Psychiatry – To find out about requirements to become an educational supervisor and local, often multidisciplinary, courses.
- NHS Trust Medical Education Department – To find out how you can get involved in teaching within the trust and courses to support this.
- Medical school – Offer courses to develop skills of those teaching and assessing undergraduates. These can open up teaching opportunities not restricted to psychiatry, e.g. facilitating case-based learning groups or communication skills training.
- University department of medical education – Some departments offer taster courses which can lead on to degree-level study.

Educational Supervisor Training

To become a named postgraduate educational or clinical supervisor or undergraduate placement lead in the United Kingdom, you need to complete training to become a recognised trainer. Your status as a trainer is overseen by the GMC and listed on the GMC register. Trainers must demonstrate competence in each of the professional standards as defined by the Academy of Medical Educators. Ensuring patient safety through good education practice is central to the standards, which span a breadth of education practice including teaching, assessment, progress monitoring, the learning environment, and professional development, both for your trainees and for you as an educator. Formal learning contributes to this process and is usually offered by your local education training board (LETB).

Degrees in Medical Education

Degrees allow you to understand the theoretical underpinnings of medical education, rather than focussing solely on practical tips. Students apply their theoretical knowledge to enhance their own teaching and are encouraged to teach and to seek feedback during the course. Furthermore, the focus is not on learning and teaching alone; it also covers other important aspects of medical education, including assessment, developing curricula, leadership, organisational learning, developing educational resources, simulation, and technology-enhanced learning.

Certificate, Diploma, and Masters Degrees

More than thirty-five universities in the United Kingdom alone offer degrees in the field of medical education. A list can be found on the Academy of Medical Educators website (www .medicaleducators.org/). Degree-level study usually starts at the Postgraduate Certificate level, though Bachelors degrees are available as intercalated BScs at some medical schools. Postgraduate Certificates require a third of the academic credit of a Master's degree (60 credits). Following completion, the student may choose to continue their study in greater depth through the diploma (a further 60 credits). Following the diploma, the Master's involves completing a piece of research in a chosen field of study and completion of a dissertation (a total of 180 credits). Full time, a Master's degree can be completed over 1 year; part-time is usually over 2–3 years.

Which Should I Choose?

Individual universities structure their degrees differently. Degree courses vary in how subjects are covered over the period of study, with compulsory and optional units, therefore it is worth considering how the topic areas covered meet your needs. For example, some focus on teaching and assessment in the certificate course, with skills more relevant to becoming a leader in education (such as curriculum development and leadership) being taught during the diploma. This may be useful if you are a clinical teaching fellow wishing to focus on improving your teaching skills, but may not meet your needs if you have just been appointed as director of medical education and want to quickly acquire relevant skills. Delivery method (face-to-face or online), assessments, and deadlines for completion will also influence your choice.

Funding your Studies

Speak to your local university, school of psychiatry, medical education department, or employer about scholarships, study budgets, and other funds to cover fees. Some universities work in partnership with training programmes to reduce costs of courses for trainees. If your role sees you supervising many medical students, it is well worth speaking to the medical education department in your trust as they may be able to offer you funding from the Medical Undergraduate Tariff (MUT), which is a payment made by the university to the NHS trust for hosting the students. Some jobs also include funding to complete a medical education degree (e.g. a clinical teaching fellow post).

Beyond Masters Level Study

If you wish to take your medical education studies further, it is possible to complete a Doctor of Education (EdD), Doctor of Medicine (MD), or Doctor of Philosophy (PhD) in education. EdDs have a larger taught component and are open to educationalists from all backgrounds, rather than concentrating on medical education. This means the taught component may focus more on school-aged education rather than the university level and beyond. MDs and PhDs involve some training (e.g. in research methodology), and are primarily research based. These involve two or three years of full-time study and are targeted towards people who may wish to pursue an academic (research) career in medical education. Funded PhDs are advertised online (e.g. findaphd.com or jobs.ac.uk). These may come with a small stipend, but this is unlikely to match your doctor's wage! For a comparable salary it is possible to apply for grant funding with a supervisor for your PhD.

Box 8.3.1 What Value do Such Courses Have?

- **Become a more confident teacher:** Understanding how to structure teaching and receiving feedback from knowledgeable others about your teaching can build confidence and help you inspire future generations of doctors.
- **Help your students learn:** Thinking about how students learn, and how you can teach in different environments, will help you make your teaching more effective. In turn, better learning means better patient care for our patient population in the future.
- **Get creative:** Understanding educational theory allows you the freedom to develop new and innovative ways to teach in an educationally informed way.
- **Take on new roles:** You may have little understanding of how assessments are developed, curricula structured, learning materials created, or medical education led and governed. Understanding the key tenets to success in these areas will help you get more meaningfully involved in these aspects of education and take on leadership roles.
- **Develop the field:** Medical education research is becoming increasingly rigorous, leading to a better evidence base. Asking and answering relevant research questions through education research allows you to develop your understanding of how to teach doctors, with potentially far-reaching effects for students, healthcare professionals, and patients.

Summary

Medical education courses offer the opportunity to develop your skills and ensure your learners get the most out of their learning opportunity and feel inspired. Many courses are free or low cost and open opportunities for educational roles within the medical school. Some educational roles (e.g. educational supervisor for trainees) require certain training to be completed. Degree courses allow you to develop a broader and deeper understanding of the field and are particularly useful if you would like education to be an important part of your career. Although they can be pricy, funding is often available to contribute to or cover the fees.

Index

Printed in the United States
by Baker & Taylor Publisher Services